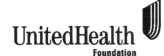

UnitedHealth Foundation
P.O. Box 1459 Minneapolis, MN 55440-1459

August, 2002

Dear Colleague,

Good clinicians understand that medical care must be based on the skillful use of scientifically valid and evidence-based information. This is why, for several years, the UnitedHealth Foundation has provided physicians and other health professionals with the BMJ's landmark publication *Clinical Evidence*. *Clinical Evidence* is the international source of the best available evidence for effective health care, and it benefits from considerable input by clinical experts from the United States in addition to others throughout the world. Traditionally it has provided easy access to the most up to date information on what is proven to work in a broad spectrum of clinical disciplines, including mental health.

As the volume of evidence-based literature and guidance in mental health has expanded over the years, the BMJ determined that a special edition devoted to mental health topics was appropriate and possible. As such, they have produced this new edition of *Clinical Evidence* entitled *Clinical Evidence Mental Health*. We at UnitedHealth Foundation are pleased to provide you with this important tool to support you in providing the best possible clinical care to your patients. In addition to this printed version of *Clinical Evidence Mental Health*, you are provided free online access to the complete text of *Clinical Evidence* that covers topics such as cardiovascular disorders; child health; digestive system disorders; ear, nose, and throat disorders; endocrine disorders; infectious diseases; kidney disorders; men's health; musculoskeletal disorders; neurological disorders; oral health; poisoniwng; sleep disorders; and women's health. To make use of this feature go to www.clinicalevidence.com. Once there, register as a recipient of UHF distribution.

Our goal at the UnitedHealth Foundation is to provide support for the medical decisions that lead to the best possible health care for the American people. We think that the new edition will assist you in providing the quality medical care that meets the high standards for which we all strive.

Sincerely,

Bill McGuire

William W. McGuire, M.D.
Chairman
UnitedHealth Foundation

clinical
evidence

Mental health

The international source of the best available evidence for effective health care

BMJ
Publishing
Group

Reprinted from *Clinical Evidence*, Issue 7, 2002, published by the BMJ Publishing Group

Editorial Office
BMJ Publishing Group, BMA House, Tavistock Square, London, WC1H 9JR, United Kingdom.
Tel: +44 (0)20 7387 4499 • Fax: +44 (0)20 7383 6242 • www.bmjpg.com

Subscription rates for the full *Clinical Evidence*
The complete edition of *Clinical Evidence* and *Clinical Evidence Concise* with companion CD-ROM are both published six monthly (June/December) by BMJ Publishing Group. The annual subscription rates for both publications (June, Issue 7, and December, Issue 8) are:

Personal: £75 • US$110 • Can$160
Institutional: £160 • US$240 • Can$345
Student/nurse: £35 • US$50 • Can$75

The combined rates, for both formats, are:

Personal: £110 • US$165 • Can$235
Institutional: £220 • US$330 • Can$475
Student/nurse: £60 • US$90 • Can$130

All individual subscriptions (personal, student, nurse) include online access at no additional cost. Institutional subscriptions are for full print/concise version only. Institutions may purchase online site licences separately. The Publishers offer discounts for any society or organisation buying bulk quantities for their members/specific groups. For further subscription information please visit the subscription pages of our website www.clinicalevidence.com or contact Miranda Lonsdale at mlonsdale@bmjgroup.com (outside the Americas) or Diane McCabe at ussales@bmjgroup.com (North and South Americas). You may also telephone us or fax us on the following numbers:

UK and ROW Tel: +44 (0)20 7383 6270 • Fax: +44 (0)20 7383 6402
Americas Tel: +1 800 373 2897/240 646 7000 • Fax: +1 240 646 7005

Contributors
If you are interested in becoming a contributor to *Clinical Evidence* please contact us at clinicalevidence@bmjgroup.com.

Rights
For information on translation rights, please contact Daniel Raymond-Barker at draymond-barker@bmjgroup.com.

British Library Cataloguing in Publication Data
A catalogue record for this book is available from the British Library:
ISBN 0-7279-1702-1

Permission to reproduce
Please contact Josephine Woodcock at jwoodcock@bmjgroup.com when requesting permission to reprint all or part of any contribution in *Clinical Evidence* or its specialty editions.

Printed by Quebecor, Kingsport, Tennessee, USA.

Team and Advisors

Acknowledgements

The BMJ Publishing Group thanks the following people and organisations for their advice and support: The Cochrane Collaboration, and especially Iain Chalmers, Mike Clarke, Phil Alderson, Peter Langhorne and Carol Lefebvre; the NHS Centre for Reviews and Dissemination, and especially Jos Kleijnen and Julie Glanville; the NHS, and especially Tom Mann, Sir John Patteson, Ron Stamp, Veronica Fraser, Muir Gray and Ben Toth; the British National Formulary, and especially Dinesh Mehta, Eric Connor and John Martin; the Health Information Research Unit at McMaster University, and especially Brian Haynes and Ann McKibbon; the UnitedHealth Foundation, and especially Dr Reed Tuckson and Yvette Krantz; the clinicians, epidemiologists, and members of patient support groups who have acted as peer reviewers. The BMJ Publishing Group values the ongoing support it has received from the global medical community for *Clinical Evidence*. In addition to others, we wish to acknowledge the efforts of the UnitedHealth Foundation who have provided educational funding to support the wide dissemination of this valuable resource to many physicians and health professionals in the USA. It is hoped that the use of this material will continue to provide expert guidance for good patient outcome. We are grateful to the clinicians and patients who spare time to take part in focus groups, which are crucial to the development of *Clinical Evidence*. Finally, we would like to acknowledge the readers who have taken the time to send us their comments and suggestions.

Contents

Clinical Evidence Mental Health

Welcome to this collection of mental health reprints from *Clinical Evidence*, a compendium of the best available evidence to guide clinical practice in specific mental health problems. This book is aimed primarily at psychiatrists, psychologists, nurses, social workers, and all therapists working in a mental health setting.

There is sometimes a perception that an evidence-based approach is less applicable in mental health than in other areas of medicine — perhaps because of the importance of personal experience and the narrative of people with mental health problems. However, whereas other areas of medicine increasingly recognise the importance of individual experience and narrative, so it has become apparent that many clinical questions and uncertainties in mental health are best answered using the same approaches from clinical epidemiology and clinical informatics that lie behind the development of evidence-based practice in general. The goal of evidence-based practice is to integrate the best currently available evidence into clinical decision making. Evidence from randomised controlled trials and systematic reviews can best inform treatment decisions, but this evidence must be used judiciously and integrated with the values and preferences of the person with a mental health problem and their relatives.[1]

Prior to becoming the section adviser for the mental health section, I discussed the project with a number of other colleagues. Some of them suggested that the task was doomed to failure because there is far too little reliable evidence about mental health. Although this did not turn out to be the case, it also overlooks the key benefit of identifying the available evidence for specific interventions as a rational way of identifying areas in need of further research.[2] Trials in mental health tend to be short and of limited quality.[3] [4] Most drug trials are conducted by the pharmaceutical industry and are aimed more at licensing bodies than at providing reliable information on which to base clinical practice.[5]

However, there is a huge amount of evidence that can helpfully inform clinical and policy decisions. Reluctance to use available research evidence probably has many origins, including practical difficulties in accessing high quality evidence and a fear that the evidence might not support many routine practices. Here it is important to recognise that the primary goal of clinical practice is to improve patients' outcomes. Evidence-based practice is simply a tool to identify approaches that are most likely to help. Most of the time, the evidence supports routine clinical practices.[6] However, on occasions, a careful examination of the evidence will suggest that certain interventions are less securely supported than had been thought, or may even suggest that they are harmful. At other times, the evidence may suggest that certain practices should be adopted more widely.

The key to successful evidence-based practice is the availability of high quality evidence — particularly summaries of the evidence. *Clinical Evidence* provides access to reliable summaries of the current best evidence to answer specific clinical questions. Starting with the clinical question means that the evidence may often be limited. Where gaps are found then they are left as overt areas of uncertainty; however, in many of the mental health section chapters included here, substantial evidence is available to guide clinical decisions. Numerical estimates of benefits and harms of specific interventions are provided whenever possible, as these are extremely helpful in helping to work out which interventions are most likely to help and least likely to harm.

TOPIC PLANS
The creation and updating of a topic involves more than performing searches and appraising the evidence. The first, and most important step in the whole process is to identify the correct questions that need to be answered in that topic. These answerable questions are structured using the standard five elements of Population, Intervention, Comparator, Outcome and time (PICOt). Detailed questions are defined iteratively, influenced by feedback from readers, surveys of questions that arise in practice, with input from contributors, experts, peer reviewers, and members of the general public. The questions that arise in clinical practice

change with time: an initial focus on whether a novel treatment works at all (where the comparator is a placebo or no treatment) is usually replaced by questioning whether one effective treatment is "better" than another (determined by direct comparison of treatments).

Until now, the development of the questions in *Clinical Evidence* has been behind closed doors. In the future, *Clinical Evidence* will post on their website the set of questions proposed for a topic as part of a "topic plan". Readers and peer reviewers will be asked to comment on the proposed structure. The idea is similar to that of the Cochrane Collaboration who post protocols for systematic reviews within the Cochrane Library.

LAUNCH OF THE CONCISE VERSION OF CLINICAL EVIDENCE
Clinical Evidence Concise was published in July 2002. It contains all the information that is within the full paper version, but most of the detail is on an enclosed CD-ROM. The paper pages list only the categorisation table, key messages and background information.

CLINICAL EVIDENCE ON HANDHELD COMPUTERS
Clinical Evidence is available as two versions for handheld computers. The AvantGo[7] version (for Palm or Windows CE devices) has been joined by Unbound Medicine's Palm version.[8] Users can choose which sections they would like to download and how much detail they need. The free software for both handheld versions is available to download from the *Clinical Evidence* website (www.clinicalevidence.com).

NEW TRANSLATIONS OF CLINICAL EVIDENCE
Spanish[9] and Russian[10] translations of *Clinical Evidence* are now available. For more information on these and other local editions, please visit www.clinicalevidence.com.

FREE ACCESS FOR DEVELOPING COUNTRIES
Clinical Evidence online is now available free or at significantly reduced cost to developing countries as part of an initiative spearheaded by the World Health Organization and the BMJ. Details of which countries are included in this offer, and how to receive content, are available from the *Clinical Evidence* website.

EVIDENCE-BASED MEDICINE SKILLS: NEW MATERIALS TO SUPPORT WORKSHOPS
Interpretation of evidence can be performed at many levels.

The simplest approach is to be a user of conclusions — someone who acts on the concrete information that drug A is effective and that drug B is not. One problem with this approach is that the conclusions have to be applied in the form they are received — tailoring conclusions to particular people is difficult.

The most detailed approach would be for an individual to identify important clinical questions in a specific context, perform searches and appraisals, integrate the evidence and then formulate the conclusions that guide treatment for particular patients. Very few health carers have the time or inclination to work routinely at this deep level.

Between these extremes lies the evidence user: a health carer who knows enough about the evidence to regenerate conclusions that are adapted to each individual. Someone who knows, for example, that NNTs (numbers needed to treat) usually vary with changes in baseline risk, with co-morbidity, and for treatments of different durations. Knowing alone is insufficient, for evidence users need to have enough skill and confidence to handle the concepts during conversation. There are many barriers to answering clinical questions.[11] One barrier is that health carers need to feel confident about their own ability to understand and manipulate the terms used in evidence-based medicine.

The development of skills and confidence is promoted by learning in small groups. There are now many excellent courses in evidence-based medicine, and many fortunate health carers have access to these courses. Materials to support such courses will be made freely available from the *Clinical Evidence* website. A number of PowerPoint presentations are now available. *Clinical Evidence* has also commissioned materials to support a 1 day interactive course on the application of evidence-based health care in clinical practice. This content has been specially written by Bazian Ltd (a specialist provider of evidence-based medicine).[12] All these materials can now be downloaded freely from the *Clinical Evidence* website (www.clinicalevidence.com).

HARMS: INADEQUATELY REPORTED IN RCTS

Information about harms is often more difficult to integrate than information about benefits.[13] Most controlled trials are designed to investigate benefits. Many either fail to document harms or present the information in a form that is difficult to analyse or interpret. When drugs are licensed they may have been used clinically in only a few thousand people; the absence of documented harms is not strong evidence that harms will not be discovered in the years after licensing.

Clinical Evidence recognises that the evidence about harms is often weaker than that about benefits. In an attempt to correct for this bias, *Clinical Evidence* has lowered the threshold for evidence to be included in the harms section. The policy is to include reports of harms that are included in the systematic reviews (or in individual RCTs if there is no systematic review) in the benefits section. *Clinical Evidence* cross refers to evidence about harms in other populations of people, on the assumption that harms are more likely than benefits to generalise across different subgroups of people. Much of the evidence for harms comes from observational studies ranging from prospective controlled cohort studies to case reports, and these are included when the harm is serious or when there is good corroborating evidence that the harm can be attributed to the treatment.

For the online version of *Clinical Evidence* the aim is to include links to external sources (e.g. the *British National Formulary* at www.bnf.org) for topics where the evidence we provide from systematic reviews and RCTs provides an incomplete and potentially misleading description of harms.

The reporting of harms requires more research and development. *Clinical Evidence* will explore the potential to provide links to other third party formularies, to improve specific searches for harms, and to liaise with other groups who are working in this area. Proposals for improved reporting will be presented on the *Clinical Evidence* website (www.clinicalevidence.com).

FEEDBACK

If you disagree with any of the material, think that important evidence has been missed, or if you have suggestions for new questions or improvements then please let us know (CEfeedback@bmjgroup.com). Thanks to all who have sent in suggestions.

REFERENCES

1. Sackett DL, Rosenberg WM, Gray JA, Haynes RB, Richardson WS. Evidence Based Medicine: what it is and what it isn't. *BMJ* 1996;312:71–72.
2. Geddes J. Asking structured and focused clinical questions: essential first step of evidence-based practice. *Evid Based Ment Health* 1999;2:35–36.
3. Johnson AL. Clinical trials in psychiatry. *Psychol Med* 1983;13:1–8.
4. Thornley B, Adams C. Content and quality of 2000 trials in schizophrenia over 50 years. *BMJ* 1998;317:1181–1184.
5. Geddes JR. Prevention of relapse in schizophrenia. *N Engl J Med* 2002;346:56–58.
6. Geddes JR, Game D, Jenkins NE, Peterson LA, Pottinger GR, Sackett DL. What proportion of primary psychiatric interventions are based on randomised evidence? *Qual Health Care* 1996;5:215–217
7. http://www.avantgo.com
8. http://www.unboundmedicine.com/cogniq.htm
9. Evidencia Clinica. Barcelona, Spain: Asociacion Colaboracion Cochrane Iberoamericana, Legis, 2002.
10. Clinical Evidence. Moscow, Russia: Media Sphera Publishing Group, 2002.
11. Ely JW, Osheroff JA, Ebell MH, et al. Obstacles to answering doctors' questions about patient care with evidence: qualitative study. *BMJ* 2002;324:710–713.
12. http://www.bazian.com
13. Derry S, Loke YK, Aronson JK. Incomplete evidence: the inadequacy of databases in tracing published adverse drug reactions in clinical trials. *BMC Medical Research Methodology* 2001;1:7 (http://www.biomedcentral.com/1471-2288/1/7).

John Geddes
Section Advisor for Mental Health
Senior Clinical Research Fellow/Honorary Consultant Psychiatrist

About Clinical Evidence

The inspiration for *Clinical Evidence* came in a phone call in 1995. Tom Mann and his colleagues at the NHS Executive asked the BMJ Publishing Group to explore the possibility of developing an evidence "formulary" along the lines of the *British National Formulary*. They recognised that clinicians were under increasing pressure to keep up-to-date and to base their practice more firmly on evidence, but that few had the necessary time or skills to do this. Their idea was to provide a pocket book containing concise and regularly updated summaries of the best available evidence on clinical interventions. However, they didn't think that the NHS could develop such a formulary itself. "It would be marvellous", said Tom Mann, "if somebody would just do it". A small team at the BMJ set to work to produce a pilot version of what was then called the *Clinical Effectiveness Directory*.

Since that pilot, a great deal has changed. In collaboration with the American College of Physicians—American Society of Internal Medicine, we convened an international advisory board, held focus groups of clinicians, talked to patient support groups, and adopted countless good ideas from early drafts by our contributors. Throughout we have kept in mind an equation set out by Slawson et al.[1] This states that the usefulness of any source of information is equal to its relevance, multiplied by its validity, divided by the work required to extract the information. In order to be as useful as possible, we aimed for high relevance, high validity, and low work in terms of the reader's time and effort. We also kept in mind principles of transparency and explicitness. Readers needed to understand where our information came from and how it was assembled.

A UNIQUE RESOURCE

Clinical Evidence joins a growing number of sources of evidence-based information for clinicians. But it has several features that make it unique.

- Its contents are driven by questions rather than by the availability of research evidence. Rather than start with the evidence and summarise what is there, we have tried to identify important clinical questions, and then to search for and summarise the best available evidence to answer them.
- It identifies but does not try to fill important gaps in the evidence. In a phrase used by Jerry Osheroff, who has led much of the recent research on clinicians' information needs,[2] *Clinical Evidence* presents the dark as well as the light side of the moon. We feel that it will be helpful for clinicians to know when their uncertainty stems from gaps in the evidence rather than gaps in their own knowledge.
- It is updated every 6 months in print and monthly online. *Clinical Evidence* is also available as a Concise pocketbook with companion CD-ROM.
- It specifically aims not to make recommendations. We feel that simply summarising the evidence will make it more widely useful. The experience of the clinical practice guideline movement has shown that it is nearly impossible to make recommendations that are appropriate in every situation. Differences in individual patients' baseline risks and preferences, and in the local availability of interventions, will always mean that the evidence must be individually interpreted rather than applied across the board. *Clinical Evidence* provides the raw material for developing locally applicable clinical practice guidelines, and for clinicians and patients to make up their own minds on the best course of action. We supply the evidence, you make the decisions.

COMPLEMENTARY BUT DIFFERENT

We are often asked how *Clinical Evidence* differs from two other high quality sources of evidence-based information: The *Cochrane Library*; and the evidence-based journals *ACP Journal Club*, *Evidence-Based Medicine*, *Evidence-Based Mental Health*, and *Evidence-Based Nursing*.

Clinical Evidence is complementary to but different from the work of the Cochrane Collaboration, which produces and publishes high quality systematic reviews of controlled trials.[3] Clinical Evidence has been called the friendly front end of the Cochrane Library, because it takes this and other, high quality information, and pulls it together in one place in a concise format. Many of our advisors and contributors are active members of the Cochrane Collaboration, and we are exploring closer ties between Clinical Evidence and the Collaboration in the way the evidence is searched for, summarised, and accessed by users.

Clinical Evidence is also complementary to but different from the evidence-based journals, which select and abstract the best and most clinically relevant articles as they appear in the world's medical literature. Together these journals form a growing archive of high quality abstracts of individual articles. Clinical Evidence takes a different approach. It begins not with the journals but with clinical questions. It is able to answer some. For others it simply reports that no good evidence was found.

DRUG NAMES
Clinical Evidence aims to present information on therapeutic drugs in a format that is relevant for an international audience. Only the generic or non-proprietary names of drugs rather that the brand names of drugs are used in Clinical Evidence, with a few exceptions where the brand name has become the commonly used name in clinical practice, for example EMLA cream (lidocaine-prilocaine). Difficulties arise when different names for the same drug are used in different parts of the world. The recommended International Name (rINN) or proposed International Name (pINN) is used where possible. Where an international name for a therapeutic drug is not available (e.g. aspirin) the most common name has been used. We have included a table of the drug names used in Clinial Evidence with the equivalent UK and US names.

A WORK IN PROGRESS
Clinical Evidence is an evolving project. We knew before we started that we were undertaking an enormous task, but the more we worked the more we realised its enormity. We recognise that there is some mismatch between what we aim eventually to achieve and what we have achieved so far. Although we have made every effort to ensure that the searches are thorough and that the appraisals of studies are objective (see Searching and Appraising the literature, p xvii), we will inevitably have missed some important studies. In order not to make unjustified claims about the accuracy of the information, we use phrases such as "we found no systematic review" rather than "there is no systematic review". In order to be as explicit as possible about the methods used for each contribution, we have asked each set of contributors to provide a brief methods section, describing the searches that were performed and how individual studies were selected.

UPDATING AND EXPANDING CLINICAL EVIDENCE
Our expectation is that Clinical Evidence will evolve rapidly in its early years. Indeed, it is already becoming a family of products, appearing in different formats and languages for different audiences. In particular, Clinical Evidence will evolve in response to the needs of clinicians. We have tried hard to anticipate those needs (not least by involving clinicians at every stage), but it is only when people begin to use Clinical Evidence in daily practice that we can know how best to develop it. That's why your feedback is so important to us, and we are arranging for various ways to evaluate the product.

REFERENCES
1. Slawson DC, Shaughnessy AF, Bennett JH. Becoming a medical information master: feeling good about not knowing everything. J Fam Pract 1994;38:505–513.
2. Ely JW, Osheroff JA, Ebell MJ, et al. Analysis of questions asked by family doctors regarding patient care. BMJ 1999; 319:358–361. http://hiru.mcmaster.ca/cochrane/default.htm.

A guide to the text

SUMMARY PAGE
The summary page for each topic presents the questions addressed, some key messages, and a list of the interventions covered, categorised according to whether they have been found to be effective or not. We have developed the categories of effectiveness from one of the Cochrane Collaboration's first and most popular products, *A guide to effective care in pregnancy and childbirth*.[1] The categories we now use are explained in the table below:

TABLE	Categorisation of treatment effects in *Clinical Evidence*
Beneficial	Interventions for which effectiveness has been demonstrated by clear evidence from RCTs, and for which expectation of harms is small compared with the benefits.
Likely to be beneficial	Interventions for which effectiveness is less well established than for those listed under "beneficial".
Trade off between benefits and harms	Interventions for which clinicians and patients should weigh up the beneficial and harmful effects according to individual circumstances and priorities.
Unknown effectiveness	Interventions for which there are currently insufficient data or data of inadequate quality.
Unlikely to be beneficial	Interventions for which lack of effectiveness is less well established than for those listed under "likely to be ineffective or harmful".
Likely to be ineffective or harmful	Interventions ineffectiveness or harmfulness has been demonstrated by clear evidence.

Fitting interventions into these categories is not always straightforward. For one thing, the categories represent a mix of several hierarchies: the level of benefit (or harm), the level of evidence (RCT or observational data), and the level of certainty around the finding (represented by the confidence interval). Another problem is that much of the evidence that is most relevant to clinical decisions relates to comparisons between different interventions rather than to comparison with placebo or no intervention. Where necessary, we have indicated the comparisons in brackets. A third problem is that interventions may have been tested, or found to be effective, in only one group of people, such as those at high risk of an outcome. Again, we have indicated this where possible. But perhaps most difficult of all has been trying to maintain consistency across different topics. We are working on refining the criteria for putting interventions under each category.

Interventions that cannot be tested in an RCT (perhaps because of ethical or practical reasons) are sometimes cited in the categorisation table, but they are always identified clearly with an asterix (for example, oxygen in severe acute asthma).

NEGATIVE FINDINGS
A surprisingly hard aspect to get right is the reporting of negative findings. As we have had to keep reminding ourselves, saying that there is no good evidence that a treatment works is not the same as saying that the treatment doesn't work. In trying to get this right, we may have erred too much on the side of caution; when in doubt we have changed summary phrases from, for example, "the review found no difference", to "the review found no evidence of a

difference". We recognise that to get this right, we need a better handle on the power of individual systematic reviews and trials to demonstrate statistically significant differences between groups, and better information on what constitutes clinically important differences in the major outcomes for each intervention. In the meantime, we hope that the text makes a clear distinction between lack of benefit and lack of evidence of benefit.

OUTCOMES
Clinical Evidence focuses on outcomes that matter to patients, meaning those that patients themselves are aware of, such as symptom severity, quality of life, survival, disability, walking distance, and live birth rate. We are less interested in proxy outcomes such as blood lipid concentrations, blood pressure, or ovulation rates. Each topic includes a list of the main patient oriented outcomes, and where possible describes how these are measured. We have for the moment decided not to address the vexed question of what constitutes a clinically important change in an outcome, but we would welcome any suggestions.

EFFECTS, NOT EFFECTIVENESS
A key aim of *Clinical Evidence* is to emphasise the important trade offs between advantages and disadvantages of different treatment options. We therefore talk about the effects of interventions, both positive and negative, rather than the effectiveness, and for each question or intervention option we present data on benefits and harms under separate headings.

HARMS
"Harms" include adverse effects of treatment and inconvenience to the patient. Finding good evidence on harms of treatments is not easy. Ideally these would come from RCTs, but many trials are not sufficiently large or long term to capture rarer or more distant events, and many do not adequately report adverse effects. We have asked contributors to keep the negative effects of interventions in mind at all times. Where good evidence is available, we indicate the frequency of adverse effects. However, because RCTs are not reliable sources of evidence about harms, and because of the principle that a physician should strive to do no harm, we also include weaker forms of evidence about harms.

DRUG INFORMATION
We make no systematic attempt to provide information on drug dosages, formulations, indications, and contraindications. For this information, we refer readers to their national drug formularies. Drug dosages are included when a question explores the relative effects of different doses.

INFORMATION ON COST
We have decided not to include information on the cost or cost effectiveness of interventions. This is not because we believe cost to be unimportant, but because the question of what constitutes good evidence on cost is much disputed and because costs vary greatly both within and between countries. However, we believe that it will become increasingly untenable for clinicians to act without paying attention to resources. Future companion publications of *Clinical Evidence* may provide relevant information on costs.

NUMERICAL DATA
Whenever possible, data are presented in the same form as in the original studies. However, sometimes we have changed the units or type of information in an attempt to present the results in a systematic and easily interpretable form.

AN INTERNATIONAL APPROACH TO THE EVIDENCE
Clinical Evidence takes an international approach to the evidence. This means including drugs that are not licensed in some countries. It also means keeping in mind the practicalities of

treating people in rich as well as poorer countries, by covering interventions even if they have been superseded (for example, single drug treatment for HIV infection as opposed to three drug treatment).

COMPETING INTERESTS
In line with the *BMJ*'s policy,[2] our aim is not to try to eliminate conflicts of interest but to make them explicit so that readers can judge for themselves what influence, if any, these may have had on the contributors' interpretation of the evidence. We therefore ask all contributors to let us know about any potential competing interests, and we append any that are declared to the end of the contribution. Where the contributor gives no competing interests, we record "none declared". Correction of an important error

HOW TO USE THE INFORMATION IN CLINICAL EVIDENCE
The type of information contained in *Clinical Evidence* is necessary but not sufficient for the provision of effective, high quality health care. It is intended as an aid to clinical decision making, to be used in conjunction with other important sources of information. These other sources include estimates of people's baseline risk of a condition or outcome based on history, physical examination and clinical investigations; individual preferences; economic arguments; availability of treatments; and local expertise.

Some guidance on how to apply research evidence in practice is available on our website (www.clinicalevidence.com) and in appendix 2.

REFERENCES
1. Enkin M, Keirse M, Renfrew M, et al. *A guide to effective care in pregnancy and childbirth*. Oxford: Oxford University Press, 1998.
2. Smith R. Beyond conflict of interest. *BMJ* 1998;317:219–292.

How Clinical Evidence is put together

The summaries in *Clinical Evidence* result from a rigorous process aimed at ensuring that the information they contain is both reliable and relevant to clinical practice.

SELECTING TOPICS
Clinical Evidence aims to cover common or important clinical conditions seen in primary and hospital care. To decide which conditions to cover in the first few issues, we reviewed national data on consultation rates, morbidity and mortality, and took advice from generalist clinicians and patient groups. Our website (www.clinicalevidence.com) provides a list of conditions that we are planning to cover in future issues. Further suggestions are welcome.

SELECTING THE QUESTIONS
The questions in *Clinical Evidence* concern the benefits and harms of preventative and therapeutic interventions, with emphasis on outcomes that matter to patients. Questions are selected for their relevance to clinical practice by section advisors and contributors, in collaboration with primary care clinicians and patient groups. Each new issue of *Clinical Evidence* will include new questions as well as updates of existing questions. Readers can suggest new clinical questions using the feedback slips to be found at the back of the book and on the *Clinical Evidence* website (www.clinicalevidence.com), or by writing directly to *Clinical Evidence*.

SEARCHING AND APPRAISING THE LITERATURE
For each question, the literature is searched using the Cochrane Library, Medline, Embase and, occasionally, other electronic databases, looking first for good systematic reviews of RCTs; then for good RCTs published since the search date of the review. Where we find no good recent systematic reviews, we search for individual RCTs. The date of the search is recorded in the methods section for each topic. Of the studies that are identified in the search, we select and summarise only a small proportion. The selection is done by critically appraising the abstracts of the studies identified in the search, a task performed independently by information scientists using validated criteria similar to those of Sackett et al[1] and Jadad.[2,3] Where the search identifies more than one or two good reviews or trials, we select those we judge to be the most robust or relevant, using the full text of the article. Where we identify few or no good reviews or trials, we include other studies but highlight their limitations. Contributors, who are chosen for their expertise in the field and their skills in epidemiology, are asked to review our selection of studies, and to justify any additions or exclusions they wish to make.

Our search strategy and critical appraisal criteria are available on our website (www.clinicalevidence.com).

SUMMARISING THE EVIDENCE, PEER REVIEW, AND EDITING
The contributors summarise the evidence relating to each question. Each topic is then peer reviewed by the section advisors and by at least three external expert clinicians. The revised text is then extensively edited by editors with clinical and epidemiological training, and data are checked against the original study reports.

REFERENCES
1. Sackett DL, Haynes RB, Guyatt GH, Tugwell P. *Clinical Epidemiology: A basic science for clinical medicine*. 2nd ed. Boston: Little Brown, 1991.
2. Jadad A. Assessing the quality of RCTs: Why, what, how and by whom? In: Jadad A, ed. *Randomised Controlled Trials*. London: BMJ Books, 1998:45—60.
3. Jadad AR, Moore RA, Carroll D, Jenkinson C, et al. Assessing the quality of reports of randomized clinical trials: is blinding necessary? *Control Clin Trials* 1996;17:1—12.

Feedback and Error Correction

Despite the extensive peer review and quality checks, we expect that the text will contain some errors and inconsistencies. Please let us know if you find any errors, either by using the comment card at the back of the book or by emailing us at CEfeedback@bmjgroup.com.

Errors are graded as minor, moderate, and major based on an assessment of their potential impact. All errors are corrected in the next printed issue of *Clinical Evidence*. Anything other than a minor error is immediately corrected in the text displayed on our website (www.clinicalevidence.com) and a list of errors corrected is available. Any major errors are highlighted on the log-in page of the website.

If you wish to be notified automatically by e-mail of any corrections and updates, then register for the *Clinical Evidence* alerting service on our website. If you are using the information in *Clinical Evidence* to guide your clinical practice then it is essential to register so that you can remain as up-to-date as possible.

Absolute risk (AR) The probability that an individual will experience the specified outcome during a specified period. It lies in the range 0 to 1, or is expressed as a percentage. In contrast to common usage, the word "risk" may refer to adverse events (such as myocardial infarction) or desirable events (such as cure).

Absolute risk increase (ARI) The absolute difference in risk between the experimental and control groups in a trial. It is used when the risk in the experimental group exceeds the risk in the control group, and is calculated by subtracting the AR in the control group from the AR in the experimental group. This figure does not give any idea of the proportional increase between the two groups: for this, relative risk (RR) is needed (see below).

Absolute risk reduction (ARR) The absolute difference in risk between the experimental and control groups in a trial. It is used when the risk in the control group exceeds the risk in the experimental group, and is calculated by subtracting the AR in the experimental group from the AR in the control group. This figure does not give any idea of the proportional reduction between the two groups: for this, relative risk (RR) is needed (see below).

Allocation concealment A method used to prevent selection bias by concealing the allocation sequence from those assigning participants to intervention groups. Allocation concealment prevents researchers from (unconsciously or otherwise) influencing which intervention group each participant is assigned to.

Applicability The application of the results from clinical trials to individual people. A randomised trial only provides direct evidence of causality within that specific trial. It takes an additional logical step to apply this result to a specific individual. Individual characteristics will affect the outcome for this person.

Baseline risk The risk of the event occurring without the active treatment. Estimated by the baseline risk in the control group.

Bias Systematic deviation of study results from the true results, because of the way(s) in which the study is conducted.

Blinding/blinded A trial is fully blinded if all the people involved are unaware of the treatment group to which trial participants are allocated until after the interpretation of results. This includes trial participants and everyone involved in administering treatment or recording trial results.

Block randomisation Randomisation by a pattern to produce the required number of people in each group.

Case control study A study design that examines a group of people who have experienced an event (usually an adverse event) and a group of people who have not experienced the same event, and looks at how exposure to suspect (usually noxious) agents differed between the two groups. This type of study design is most useful for trying to ascertain the cause of rare events, such as rare cancers.

Case series Analysis of series of people with the disease (there is no comparison group in case series).

Clinically significant A finding that is clinically important. Here, "significant" takes its everyday meaning of "important" (compared with statistically significant; see below). Where the word "significant" or "significance" is used without qualification in the text, it is being used in its statistical sense.

Cluster randomisation A cluster randomised study is one in which a group of participants are randomised to the same intervention together. Examples of cluster randomisation include allocating together people in the same village, hospital, or school. If the results are then analysed by individuals rather than the group as a whole bias can occur.

Cohort study A non-experimental study design that follows a group of people (a cohort), and then looks at how events differ among people within the group. A study that examines a cohort, which differs in respect to exposure to some suspected risk factor (e.g. smoking), is useful for trying to ascertain whether exposure is likely to cause specified events (e.g. lung cancer). Prospective cohort studies (which track participants forward in time) are more reliable than retrospective cohort studies.

Completer analysis Analysis of data from only those participants who remained at the end of the study. Compare with intention to treat analysis, which uses data from all participants who enrolled (see below).

Confidence interval (CI) The 95% confidence interval (or 95% confidence limits) would include 95% of results from studies of the same size and design in the same population. This is close but not identical to saying that the true size of the effect (never exactly known) has a 95% chance of falling within the confidence interval. If the 95% confidence interval for a relative risk (RR) or an odds ratio (OR) crosses 1, then this is taken as no evidence of an effect. The practical advantages of a confidence interval (rather than a P value) is that they present the range of likely effects.

Controls In a randomised controlled trial (RCT), controls refer to the participants in its comparison group. They are allocated either to placebo, no treatment, or a standard treatment.

Crossover randomised trial A trial in which participants receive one treatment and have outcomes measured, and then receive an alternative treatment and have outcomes measured again. The order of treatments is randomly assigned. Sometimes a period of no treatment is used before the trial starts and in between the treatments (washout periods) to minimise interference between the treatments (carry over effects). Interpretation of the results from crossover randomised controlled trials (RCTs) can be complex.

Cross sectional study A study design that involves surveying a population about an exposure, or condition, or both, at one point in time. It can be used for assessing prevalence of a condition in the population.

Effect size (standardised mean differences) In the medical literature, effect size is used to refer to a variety of measures of treatment effect. In *Clinical Evidence* it refers to a standardised mean difference: a statistic for combining continuous variables (such as pain scores or height), from different scales, by dividing the difference between two means by an estimate of the within group standard deviation.

Event The occurrence of a dichotomous outcome that is being sought in the study (such as myocardial infarction, death, or a four-point improvement in pain score).

Experimental study A study in which the investigator studies the effect of intentionally altering one or more factors under controlled conditions.

Factorial design A factorial design attempts to evaluate more than one intervention compared with control in a single trial, by means of multiple randomisations.

False negative A person with the target condition (defined by the gold standard) who has a negative test result.

False positive A person without the target condition (defined by the gold standard) who has a positive test result.

Fixed effects The "fixed effects" model of meta-analysis assumes, often unreasonably, that the variability between the studies is exclusively because of a random sampling variation around a fixed effect (see random effects below).

Hazard ratio (HR) Broadly equivalent to relative risk (RR); useful when the risk is not constant with respect to time. It uses information collected at different times. The term is typically used in the context of survival over time. If the HR is 0.5 then the relative risk of dying in one group is half the risk of dying in the other group.

Heterogeneity In the context of meta-analysis, heterogeneity means dissimilarity between studies. It can be because of the use of different statistical methods (statistical heterogeneity), or evaluation of people with different characteristics, treatments or outcomes (clinical heterogeneity). Heterogeneity may render pooling of data in meta-analysis unreliable or inappropriate.

Homogeneity Similarity (see heterogeneity above).

Incidence The number of new cases of a condition occurring in a population over a specified period of time.

Intention to treat analysis Analysis of data for all participants based on the group to which they were randomised and not based on the actual treatment they received.

Likelihood ratio The ratio of the probability that an individual with the target condition has a specified test result to the probability that an individual without the target condition has the same specified test result.

Meta-analysis A statistical technique that summarises the results of several studies in a single weighted estimate, in which more weight is given to results of studies with more events and sometimes to studies of higher quality.

Morbidity Rate of illness but not death.

Mortality Rate of death.

Negative likelihood ratio (NLR) The ratio of the probability that an individual with the target condition has a negative test result to the probability that an individual without the target condition has a negative test result. This is the same as the ratio (1-sensitivity/specificity).

Negative predictive value (NPV) The chance of not having a disease given a negative test result (not to be confused with specificity, which is the other way round; see below).

Not significant/non-significant (NS) In *Clinical Evidence*, not significant means that the observed difference, or a larger difference, could have arisen by chance with a probability of more than 1/20 (i.e. 5%), assuming that there is no underlying difference. This is not the same as saying there is no effect, just that this experiment does not provide convincing evidence of an effect. This could be because the trial was not powered to detect an effect that does exist, because there was no effect, or because of the play of chance.

Number needed to harm (NNH) One measure of treatment harm. It is the average number of people from a defined population you would need to treat with a specific intervention for a given period of time to cause one additional adverse outcome. NNH can be calculated as 1/ARI. In *Clinical Evidence*, these are usually rounded downwards.

Number needed to treat (NNT) One measure of treatment effectiveness. It is the number of people you would on average need to treat with a specific intervention for a given period of time to prevent one additional adverse outcome or achieve one additional beneficial outcome. NNT can be calculated as 1/ARR (see appendix 2). In *Clinical Evidence*, NNTs are usually rounded upwards.

NNT for a meta-analysis Absolute measures are useful at describing the effort required to obtain a benefit, but are limited because they are influenced by both the treatment and also by the baseline risk of the individual. If a meta-analysis includes individuals with a range of baseline risks, then no single NNT will be applicable to the people in that meta-analysis, but a single relative measure (odds ratio or relative risk) may be applicable if there is no heterogeneity. In *Clinical Evidence*, an NNT is provided for meta-analysis, based on a combination of the summary odds ratio (OR) and the mean baseline risk observed in average of the control groups.

Odds The odds of an event happening is defined as the probability that an event will occur, expressed as a proportion of the probability that the event will not occur.

Odds ratio (OR) One measure of treatment effectiveness. It is the odds of an event happening in the experimental group expressed as a proportion of the odds of an event happening in the control group. The closer the OR is to one, the smaller the difference in effect between the experimental intervention and the control intervention. If the OR is greater (or less) than one, then the effects of the treatment are more (or less) than those of the control treatment. Note that the effects being measured may be adverse (e.g. death or disability) or desirable (e.g. survival). When events are rare the OR is analogous to the relative risk (RR), but as event rates increase the OR and RR diverge.

Odds reduction The complement of odds ratio (1-OR), similar to the relative risk reduction (RRR) when events are rare.

Placebo A substance given in the control group of a clinical trial, which is ideally identical in appearance and taste or feel to the experimental treatment and believed to lack any disease specific effects. In the context of non-pharmacological interventions, placebo is usually referred to as sham treatments (see sham treatment below).

Positive likelihood ratio (LR+) The ratio of the probability that an individual with the target condition has a positive test result to the probability that an individual without the target condition has a positive test result. This is the same as the ratio (sensitivity/1-specificity).

Positive predictive value (PPV) The chance of having a disease given a positive test result (not to be confused with sensitivity, which is the other way round; see below).

Power A study has adequate power if it can reliably detect a clinically important difference (i.e. between two treatments) if one actually exists. The power of a study is increased when it includes more events or when its measurement of outcomes is more precise.

Pragmatic study An RCT designed to provide results that are directly applicable to normal practice (compared with explanatory trials that are intended to clarify efficacy under ideal conditions). Pragmatic RCTs recruit a population that is representative of those who are normally treated, allow normal compliance with instructions (by avoiding incentives and by using oral instructions with advice to follow manufacturers instructions), and analyse results by "intention to treat" rather than by "on treatment" methods.

Prevalence The proportion of people with a finding or disease in a given population at a given time.

Publication bias Occurs when the likelihood of a study being published varies with the results it finds. Usually, this occurs when studies that find a significant effect are more likely to be published than studies that do not find a significant effect, so making it appear from surveys of the published literature that treatments are more effective than is truly the case.

P value The probability that an observed or greater difference occurred by chance, if it is assumed that there is in fact no real difference between the effects of the interventions. If this probability is less than 1/20 (which is when the P value is less than 0.05), then the result is conventionally regarded as being "statistically significant".

Quasi randomised A trial using a method of allocating participants to different forms of care that is not truly random; for example, allocation by date of birth, day of the week, medical record number, month of the year, or the order in which participants are included in the study (e.g. alternation).

Random effects The "random effects" model assumes a different underlying effect for each study and takes this into consideration as an additional source of variation, which leads to somewhat wider confidence intervals than the fixed effects model. Effects are assumed to be randomly distributed, and the central point of this distribution is the focus of the combined effect estimate (see fixed effects above).

Randomised controlled trial (RCT) A trial in which participants are randomly assigned to two or more groups: at least one (the experimental group) receiving an intervention that is being tested and an other (the comparison or control group) receiving an alternative treatment or placebo. This design allows assessment of the relative effects of interventions.

Regression analysis Given data on a dependent variable and one or more independent variables, regression analysis involves finding the "best" mathematical model to describe or predict the dependent variable as a function of the independent variable(s). There are several regression models that suit different needs. Common forms are linear, logistic, and proportional hazards.

Relative risk (RR) The number of times more likely (RR > 1) or less likely (RR < 1) an event is to happen in one group compared with another. It is the ratio of the absolute risk (AR) for each group. It is analogous to the odds ratio (OR) when events are rare.

Relative risk increase (RRI) The proportional increase in risk between experimental and control participants in a trial.

Relative risk reduction (RRR) The proportional reduction in risk between experimental and control participants in a trial. It is the complement of the relative risk (1-RR).

Sensitivity The chance of having a positive test result given that you have a disease (not to be confused with positive predictive value [PPV], which is the other way around; see above).

Sensitivity analysis Analysis to test if results from meta-analysis are sensitive to restrictions on the data included. Common examples are large trials only, higher quality trials only, and more recent trials only. If results are consistent this provides stronger evidence of an effect and of generalisability.

Sham treatment An intervention given in the control group of a clinical trial, which is ideally identical in appearance and feel to the experimental treatment and believed to lack any disease specific effects (e.g. detuned ultrasound or random biofeedback).

Significant By convention, taken to mean statistically significant at the 5% level (see statistically significant below). This is the same as a 95% confidence interval not including the value corresponding to no effect.

Specificity The chance of having a negative test result given that you do not have a disease (not to be confused with negative predictive value [NPV], which is the other way around; see above).

Standardised mean difference (SMD) A measure of effect size used when outcomes are continuous (such as height, weight, or symptom scores) rather than dichotomous (such as death or myocardial infarction). The mean differences in outcome between the groups being studied are standardised to account for differences in scoring methods (such as pain scores). The measure is a ratio; therefore, it has no units.

Statistically significant Means that the findings of a study are unlikely to have arisen because of chance. Significance at the commonly cited 5% level ($P < 0.05$) means that the observed difference or greater difference would occur by chance in only 1/20 similar cases. Where the word "significant" or "significance" is used without qualification in the text, it is being used in this statistical sense.

Subgroup analysis Analysis of a part of the trial/meta-analysis population in which it is thought the effect may differ from the mean effect.

Systematic review A review in which specified and appropriate methods have been used to identify, appraise, and summarise studies addressing a defined question. It can, but need not, involve meta-analysis (see meta-analysis). In *Clinical Evidence*, the term systematic review refers to a systematic review of RCTs unless specified otherwise.

True negative A person without the target condition (defined by a gold standard) who has a negative test result.

True positive A person with the target condition (defined by a gold standard) who also has a positive test result.

Validity The soundness or rigour of a study. A study is internally valid if the way it is designed and carried out means that the results are unbiased and it gives you an accurate estimate of the effect that is being measured. A study is externally valid if its results are applicable to people encountered in regular clinical practice.

Weighted mean difference (WMD) A measure of effect size used when outcomes are continuous (such as symptom scores or height) rather than dichotomous (such as death or myocardial infarction). The mean differences in outcome between the groups being studied are weighted to account for different sample sizes and differing precision between studies. The WMD is an absolute figure and so takes the units of the original outcome measure.

Drug conversion list

The following information on nomenclature and brand names is provided by *Martindale: The Complete Drug Reference,* the foremost source for medicines information worldwide.[1]

Clinical Evidence name(s)*	International name(s)†	UK name(s)‡	USA name(s)§
Abecarnil	Abecarnil	—	—
Alprazolam	Alprazolam	Alprazolam	Alprazolam
Amisulpride	Amisulpride	Amisulpride	—
Amitriptyline	Amitriptyline	Amitriptyline	Amitriptyline
Aspirin	—	Aspirin	Aspirin
Brofaromine	Brofaromine	—	—
Bromazepam	Bromazepam	Bromazepam	Bromazepam
Bupropion	Bupropion	Bupropion	Bupropion
Buspirone	Buspirone	Buspirone	Buspirone
Carbamazepine	Carbamazepine	Carbamazepine	Carbamazepine
Chlorpromazine	Chlorpromazine	Chlorpromazine	Chlorpromazine
Cisapride	Cisapride	Cisapride	Cisapride
Citalopram	Citalopram	Citalopram	—
Clomipramine	Clomipramine	Clomipramine	Clomipramine
Clonidine	Clonidine	Clonidine	Clonidine
Clopenthixol decanoate	Clopenthixol decanoate	Clopenthixol decanoate	Clopenthixol decanoate
Clozapine	Clozapine	Clozapine	Clozapine
Conjugated oestrogens (equine)	—	Conjugated oestrogens	Conjugated estrogens
Cyproheptadine	Cyproheptadine	Cyproheptadine	Cyproheptadine
Desipramine	Desipramine	Desipramine	Desipramine
Dexamfetamine	Dexamfetamine	Dexamfetamine	Dextroamphetamine
Diazepam	Diazepam	Diazepam	Diazepam
Diclofenac	Diclofenac	Diclofenac	Diclofenac
Donepezil	Donepezil	Donepezil	Donepezil
Fludrocortisone	Fludrocortisone	Fludrocortisone	Fludrocortisone
Fluoxetine	Fluoxetine	Fluoxetine	Fluoxetine
Flupentixol	Flupentixol	Flupentixol	—
Fluphenazine	Fluphenazine	Fluphenazine	Fluphenazine
Fluspirilene decanoate	Fluspirilene decanoate	Fluspirilene decanoate	Fluspirilene decanoate
Fluvoxamine	Fluvoxamine	Fluvoxamine	Fluvoxamine
Galantamine	Galantamine	Galantamine	Galantamine

Clinical Evidence name(s)*	International name(s)†	UK name(s)‡	USA name(s)§
Haloperidol	Haloperidol	Haloperidol	Haloperidol
Hydrocortisone	Hydrocortisone	Hydrocortisone	Hydrocortisone
Hydroxyzine	Hydroxyzine	Hydroxyzine	Hydroxyzine
Imipramine	Imipramine	Imipramine	Imipramine
Indometacin	Indometacin	Indometacin	Indomethacin
Interferon alfa	Interferon alfa	Interferon alfa	Interferon alfa
Interferon beta	Interferon beta	Interferon beta	Interferon beta
Interferon gamma	Interferon gamma	Interferon gamma	Interferon gamma
Isocarboxazid	Isocarboxazid	Isocarboxazid	Isocarboxazid
Isoflavone	—	—	—
Lamotrigine	Lamotrigine	Lamotrigine	Lamotrigine
Lecithin	—	—	Lecithin
Lithium carbonate or Lithium citrate	—	Lithium carbonate or Lithium Citrate	Lithium carbonate or Lithium citrate
Loxapine	Loxapine	Loxapine	Loxapine
Methylphenidate	Methylphenidate	Methylphenidate	Methylphenidate
Mianserin	Mianserin	Mianserin	Mianserin
Misoprostol	Misoprostol	Misoprostol	Misoprostol
Moclobemide	Moclobemide	Moclobemide	Moclobemide
Molindone	Molindone	Molindone	Molindone
Nefazodone	Nefazodone	Nefazodone	Nefazodone
Nicotinamide adenine dinucleotide	Nadide	Nadide	Nadide
Nicotine	—	Nicotine	Nicotine
Nortriptyline	Nortriptyline	Nortriptyline	Nortriptyline
Olanzapine	Olanzapine	Olanzapine	Olanzapine
Opipramol	Opipramol	Opipramol	Opipramol
Paroxetine	Paroxetine	Paroxetine	Paroxetine
Perphenazine enanthate	Perphenazine enantate	Perphenazine enantate	Perphenazine enanthate
Phenelzine	Phenelzine	Phenelzine	Phenelzine
Physostigmine	—	Physostigmine	Physostigmine
Pimozide	Pimozide	Pimozide	Pimozide
Pipotiazine palmitate	Pipotiazine palmitate	Pipotiazine palmitate	Pipotiazine palmitate
Quetiapine	Quetiapine	Quetiapine	Quetiapine
Risperidone	Risperidone	Risperidone	Risperidone
Ritanserin	Ritanserin	Ritanserin	Ritanserin

Clinical Evidence name(s)*	International name(s)†	UK name(s)‡	USA name(s)§
Rivastigmine	Rivastigmine	Rivastigmine	Rivastigmine
Selegiline	Selegiline	Selegiline	Selegiline
Sertraline	Sertraline	Sertraline	Sertraline
Sodium valproate	Sodium valproate	Sodium valproate	Valproate sodium
Sulpiride	Sulpiride	Sulpiride	Sulpiride
Tacrine	Tacrine	Tacrine	Tacrine
Tetrazepam	Tetrazepam	Tetrazepam	—
Thioridazine	Thioridazine	Thioridazine	Thioridazine
Trazodone	Trazodone	Trazodone	Trazodone
Trifluoperazine	Trifluoperazine	Trifluoperazine	Trifluoperazine
Venlafaxine	Venlafaxine	Venlafaxine	Venlafaxine
Zimelidine	Zimelidine	Zimelidine	Zimelidine
Zinc gluconate	—	—	Zinc gluconate
Ziprasidone	Ziprasidone	Ziprasidone	Ziprasidone
Zotepine	Zotepine	Zotepine	—
Zuclopenthixol decanoate	Zuclopenthixol decanoate	Zuclopenthixol decanoate	Zuclopenthixol decanoate

*Clinical Evidence name(s): the name that appears in the Clinical Evidence index.
†International name(s): the recommended International Non-proprietary Name (rINN) or proposed International Non-proprietary Name (pINN).
‡UK name(s): the British Approved Name (BAN) or British Pharmacopoeia (BP) 2001 name.
§USA name(s): United States Formulary (USNF) 20th Edition, 2002 name or United States Pharmacopoeia (USP) 25th Edition, 2002 name.

1. Sweetman SC, Editor. Martindale: The Complete Drug Reference. 33rd edition. London: Pharmaceutical Press, 2002. See http://www.pharmpress.com or contact martindale@rpsgb.org.uk.

UK and US terms

UK / US

A

a tenth / one-tenth
acute glaucoma / acute narrow-angle glaucoma
adrenaline / epinephrine
aetiology / etiology
after effect / aftereffect
ageing / aging
allogenic / allogeneic
amenorrhoea / amenorrhea
amoebic, amoebiasis / amebic, amebiasis
anaesthesia / anesthesia
anaesthetic / anesthetic
analyse / analyze
antenatal / prenatal
antiacne / anti-acne
aortic incompetance / aortic regurgitation
apnoea / apnea
arrector / erector
artificial ventilation / artificial respiration or rescue breathing

B

bacteraemic / bacteremic
barrier cream / emollient cream
behaviour / behavior
blocked nose / stuffy nose
blueish / bluish
bow leg / bowleg
breast feed, breast feeding / breastfeed, breastfeeding
buphthalmos / congenital glaucoma
byproduct / by-product

C

caesarean section / cesarean section
callus (adj) / callous (adj) (noun is callus)
case series / case reports
casualty (first aid) / victim ("casualties", in US are usually dead)
casualty department / emergency room
channelled / channeled
chest drain / chest tube
chiropodist / podiatrist
coeliac disease / celiac disease
combined contraception pill / combination oral contraceptives

coronary heart disease / coronary artery disease
cot / crib
cotton bud / cotton swab
counselling / counseling
cranial diabetes / central diabetes
childminder / day care

D

desferrioxamine / deferoxamine
diarrhoea / diarrhea
diathermycoagulation / diathermocoagulation
disc / disk
diverticular disease / diverticulosis
Down's syndrome / Down syndrome
d-penicillamine / penicillamine
dummy / pacifier
dysaethesia / dysethesia
dysmenorrhoea / dysmenorrhea
dyspnoea / dyspnea

E

ear defenders / hearing protective devices
ear drops / eardrops
ear drum / eardrum
ear wax / earwax
end point / endpoint
energy / calories
exclude / rule out
extrinsic allergic alveolitis / hypersensitivity pneumonitis
eye drops / eyedrops

F

faeces / feces
false colour (x rays) / color-enhanced (X-rays)
feed, feeds (infant meal) / feeding, feedings
fibre / fiber
fibreoptic / fiberoptic
fibrosing alveolitis / interstitial fibrosis
fit / seizure
flexural psoriasis / inverse psoriasis
focusing errors / refractive errors

G

galactorrhoea / galactorrhea
gall stones / gallstones

gastro-oesophageal reflux disease (GORD) / gastroesophageal reflux disease (GERD)
giddiness / dizziness
gingivae / gingiva
glycaemic / glycemic
glyceryl trinitrate / nitroglycerin
gonadotrophin / gonadotropin
gonorrhoea / gonorrhea
greasy / oily
guaiphenesin / guaifenesin
gynaecomastin / gynecomastia

H

haemangiomata / hemangiomata
haemochromatosis / hemochromatosis
haemodialysis / hemodialysis
haemoglobin / hemoglobin
haemolysis / hemolysis
haemolytic / hemolytic
haemorrhage / hemorrhage
harms / risks
heat pad / heating pad
hot flushes / hot flashes
humour / humor
hyoscine hydrobromide / scopolamine hydrobromide
hypercholesterolaemia / hypercholesterolemia
hyperlipidaemia / hyperlipidemia
hypermetropia / hyperopia
hyperuricaemia / hyperuricemia
hypoglycaemia / hypoglycemia
hypoxaemia / hypoxemia
hysterosalpingogram / hydrosonography

I

indirect laryngoscopy / flexible fiberoptic laryngoscopy
information tag / emergency bracelet
interferon alpha / interferon alfa
ischaemic / ischemic

L

labour / labor
leukaemia / leukemia
localised / localized
long sight / farsightedness
looking after your back / taking care of your back
lymphoedema / lymphedema

M

menotrophin / menotropin
methohexitone / methohexital
mitozantrone / mitoxantrone
mitral incompetance / mitral regurgitation
moracizine / moricizine
mould / mold

N

naevus, nacvi / nevus, nevi
nail body / nail plate
nail root / nail matrix
named after / named for
nappy / diaper
nasendoscopy / nasal endoscopy
nasendoscope / nasal endoscope
nebuliser / nebulizer
nipple cream / moisturizing cream
non-opioid / nonopioid
non-perfumed / nonperfumed
non-smoker / nonsmoker
non-steroidal / nonsteridal
non-ulcer dyspepsia / nonulcer dyspepsia
noradrenaline / norepinephrine
norethisterone / norethindrone

O

odour / odor
oedema / edema
oesophagus / esophagus
oestrogen / estrogen
on prescription / by prescription
optician, optometrist / ophthalmologist
over sensitive / oversensitive
oxidisation / oxidation

P

painkiller / analgesic
paracetamol / acetaminophen
paralyse / paralyze
pass urine / urinate
pass wind / pass gas
pelvic floor exercises / Kegel exercises
per cent / percent
period / menstrual period, menstruation
persistent anxiety state / generalized anxiety disorder
physiotherapy / physical therapy
phlegm / sputum

pile(s) / hemorroid(s)
pilonidal sinus / pilonidal cyst
placenta praevia / placenta previa
plaster / adhesive bandage
polycythaemia / polycythemia
possetting / spitting up
premature labour / preterm labor
preventative / preventive
pre-eclampsia / preeclampsia

R
radio-opaque dye / radiopaque dye
radiotherapy / radiation therapy,
    treatment
realise / realize
re-attach / reattach
recognise / recognize
reducing diet / weight-loss diet
resolve (the disease resolves) / clears
    up, disappears, etc
ribbon gauze / nasal tampons, spongers
rifampicin / rifampin

S
sandpit / sandbox
sanitary towels / sanitary napkins
seborrhoea / seborrhea
seborrhoeic / seborrheic
semi-liquid / semiliquid
septicaemia / septicemia
severely / profoundly
short sight / nearsightedness
sickle cell anaemia / sickle-cell anemia
skin-tunnelled catheter / skin-tunneled
    venous catheter
sleep apnoea / sleep apnea
sodium cromoglycate / cromolyn sodium
sodium valproate / valproate sodium
soiling / defecation

solar keratosis / actinic keratosis
spectacles / glasses (or cycglasses)
sulphasalazine / sulfasalazine
sulphate / sulfate
sulphonamide / sulfonamide
sulphonylurca / sulfonylurca
sunbeds / sunlamps / tanning booths
suppleness / flexibility

T
tachypnoea / tachypnea
teat (bottle) / nipple (bottle as well as
    breast)
tendon hammer / reflex hammer
thalassaemia / thalassemia
threadworm(s) / pinworm(s)
though / although
thyroid tumours / thyroid nodules
tiredness / fatigue
tonometer / applantation tonometer
tonometry / applantation tonometry
trace / tracing
trainers / sneakers
tranquiliser / tranquilizer
tumour / tumor

V
venesection / phlebotomy
videocystometrogram / video
    urodynamics

W
wart paint / wart remover
waters (amniotic fluid) / water
weal / wheal
weep / ooze
wind / gas, burp

Search date April 2001

Janet Treasure and Ulrike Schmidt

INTERVENTIONS

Key Messages

- One small RCT found limited evidence that various psychotherapies were more effective than treatment as usual. One other small RCT found no significant difference between psychotherapy and dietary advice. One small RCT found a 100% withdrawal rate with dietary advice. Seven small RCTs found no overall significant differences between different psychotherapies. However, all the RCTs were small and were unlikely to have been powered to detect a difference between treatments.

- Four RCTs found no evidence that the addition of an antidepressant to treatment improved outcomes.

- Three RCTs found no evidence that cyproheptadine increased weight gain compared with placebo.

- Limited evidence from one small RCT found outpatient treatment was as effective as inpatient treatment in those individuals not so severely ill as to warrant emergency intervention.

- One small RCT found no benefit from zinc in the treatment of anorexia nervosa.

- One small RCT found no benefit from cisapride in the treatment of anorexia nervosa.

- We found no good evidence of the effect of hormonal treatment on fracture rates. One small RCT found no effect of oestrogen on bone mineral density.

- We found no RCTs to support the use of neuroleptic medication in anorexia nervosa.

DEFINITION Anorexia nervosa is characterised by a refusal to maintain weight at or above a minimally normal weight (< 85% of expected weight for age and height, or body mass index [BMI — see glossary, p 8] < 17.5 kg/m^2), or a failure to show the expected weight gain during growth. In association with this, there is often an intense fear of gaining weight, preoccupation with weight, denial of the current low weight and its adverse impact on health, and amenorrhoea. Two subtypes of anorexia nervosa, binge–purge and restricting, have been defined.[1]

INCIDENCE/ PREVALENCE A mean incidence in the general population of 19/100 000 a year in females and 2/100 000 a year in males has been estimated from 12 cumulative studies.[2] The highest rate was in female teenagers (age 13–19 years), where there were 50.8 cases/100 000 a year. A large cohort study of Swedish school children (4291 people, age 16 years) were screened by weighing and subsequent interview, and the prevalence of anorexia nervosa cases (defined using DSM-III and DSM-III-R criterita) was found to be 7/1000 for girls and 1/1000 for boys.[3] Little is known of the incidence or prevalence in Asia, South America, or Africa.

AETIOLOGY/ RISK FACTORS The aetiology of anorexia nervosa has been related to family, biological, social, and cultural factors.[4] Studies have found that anorexia nervosa is associated with a family history of anorexia nervosa (HR 11.4, 95% CI 1.1 to 89), of bulimia nervosa (adjusted HR 3.5, 955 CI 1.1 to 14),[5] depression, generalised anxiety disorder, obsessive complusive disorder, or obsessive compulsive personality disorder (adjusted RR 3.6, 95% CI 1.6 to 8).[6] A twin study estimated the heritability to be 58% (95% CI 33% to 77%), with the remaining variance apparently due to non-shared environment. However, the study was unable to completely rule out a contribution of a non-shared environment. Specific aspects of childhood temperament thought to be related include perfectionism, negative self-evaluation, and extreme compliance.[7] Perinatal factors include prematurity (OR 3.2, 95% CI 1.6 to 6.2), particularly if the baby was small for gestational age (OR 5.7, 95% CI 1.4 to 4.1).

PROGNOSIS We found no good evidence on the prognosis of people with anorexia nervosa who do not access formal medical care. A summary of treatment studies (68 studies published between 1953 and 1989, 3104 people, length of follow up 1–33 years) found that 43% of people recover completely (range 7–86%), 36% improve (range 1–69%), 20% develop a chronic eating disorder (range 0–43%), and 5% die from anorexia nervosa (range 0–21%).[8] Favourable prognostic factors include an early age at onset and a short interval between onset of symptoms and the beginning of treatment. Unfavourable prognostic factors include vomiting, bulimia, profound weight loss, chronicity, and a history of premorbid developmental or clinical abnormalities. The all cause standardised mortality ratio of eating disorders (anorexia nervosa and bulimia nervosa) has been estimated at 538, about three times higher than other psychiatric illness.[9] The average annual risk of mortality was 0.59% a year in females in 10 eating disorder populations (1322 people) with a minimum follow up of 6 years.[10] The mortality risk

We are pleased to provide you with this copy of
Clinical Evidence Mental Health.

We at UnitedHealth Foundation support you in your efforts to
provide the best quality of health care for your patients.

For more information on UnitedHealth Foundation,
please visit our website at:

www.unitedhealthfoundation.org.

Clinical Evidence Mental Health Questionnaire

As a recipient of *Clinical Evidence Mental Health* your feedback is
important to help us serve your needs. We hope you will take a
moment to answer and return this brief survey.

1 How relevant is the content of this book to your practice?
- ☐ Very useful   ☐ Somewhat useful
- ☐ Useful   ☐ Not at all useful

2 Do you find *Clinical Evidence Mental Health* easy to use?
- ☐ Yes   ☐ No

3 Has receiving *Clinical Evidence Mental Health* helped you
alter, modify or confirm any aspect of your clinical practice?
- ☐ Yes   ☐ No

4 Is the website **www.clinialevidence.com** user friendly
and easy to access?
- ☐ Yes   ☐ No   ☐ Don't Know/Didn't Use

5 Would you be interested in receiving future copies of *Clinical
Evidence Mental Health* if they are available?
- ☐ Yes   ☐ No

Name ....

Address ....

....

....

City...................................State..............................Zip....................

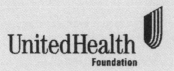

UnitedHealth
Foundation

P.O. Box 1459
Minneapolis, Minnesota 55440
www.unitedhealthfoundation.org
e-mail: ce@unitedhealthfoundation.org

Please add
Postage for
Mailing

UnitedHealth Foundation
MN008-T500
P.O. Box 1459
Minneapolis, MN 55440

UnitedHealth Foundation
Clinical Evidence
MN008-T500
P.O. Box 1459
Minneapolis, MN 55440-1459

was higher for people with lower weight and with older age at presentation. Young women with anorexia nervosa are at an increased risk of fractures later in life.[11]

AIMS
To restore physical health (weight within the normal range and no sequelae of starvation, e.g. regular menstruation, normal bone mass), normal patterns of eating and attitudes towards weight and shape, and no additional psychiatric comorbidity (e.g. depression, anxiety, obsessive compulsive disorder); to reduce the impact of the illness on social functioning and quality of life.

OUTCOMES
The most widely used measure of outcome is the Morgan and Russell scale (see glossary, p 8),[12] which includes nutritional status, menstrual function, mental state, and sexual and social adjustment. Biological outcome criteria alone such as weight (BMI or in relation to matched population weight) and menstrual function are used infrequently as outcome measures. RCTs do not usually have sufficient power or long enough follow up periods to address mortality. Other validated outcome measures used include eating symptom measures.[13–16]

METHODS
Clinical Evidence search and appraisal April 2001, and hand search of reference lists of identified reviews. To be included, an RCT had to have at least 30 people and follow up greater than 75%. Results from each of the identified trials were extracted independently by the two reviewers. Any disagreements were discussed until a consensus was reached. A systematic review (in German) was identified through direct contact with the author and is awaiting translation.[17]

QUESTION   What are the effects of treatments in anorexia nervosa?

OPTION   PSYCHOTHERAPY

One small RCT found limited evidence that various psychotherapies were more effective than treatment as usual. One other small RCT found no significant difference between psychotherapy and dietary advice. One small RCT found a 100% withdrawal rate with dietary advice. Seven small RCTs found no significant difference between different psychotherapies.

Benefits:
We found no systematic review. We found nine small RCTs. Three small RCTs of limited quality compared different psychotherapies (see glossary, p 8) versus dietary advice (see glossary, p 8) or treatment as usual (see web extra table A at www.clinicalevidence. com). All three RCTs were carried out in an outpatient setting in people with a late age of onset and long duration of illness.[18–20] The largest RCT found significant improvements in weight gain for some psychotherapies versus treatment as usual and for the number of people classified as recovered.[18] The second RCT found a significant improvement for cognitive therapy versus baseline.[20] All people treated with dietary advice withdrew from treatment and refused release of their results, making it impossible to compare the two groups. The third RCT found no difference in outcomes between the groups (see web extra table A at www.clinicalevidence.com).[19] Seven small RCTs of limited quality compared different psychotherapies. Three of these were undertaken in an outpatient

setting,[21–23] and one was carried out in an inpatient setting[24] in people with an early age of onset and short illness duration. Two of the RCTs were carried out in an outpatient setting in people with a later age of onset and longer duration of illness.[18,25] One RCT included people with early and late onset anorexia nervosa and with long and short duration of illness.[26,27] No RCT found an overall significant difference between different psychotherapies.

Harms: The acceptability of the treatment varied between RCTs. Failure to engage or early withdrawal from treatment ranged from 5–33% between RCTs (4/84 [5%];[18] 7/33 [21%];[23] 19/56 [33%];[24] 8/54 [14%];[26] 7/43 [16%][21]), but this may have been caused by different methods of case ascertainment. The number of people admitted for inpatient treatment (see glossary, p 8) also varied between RCTs, ranging from 0–36% (12/84 [14%];[18] 3/30 [10%];[19] 0/30 [0%];[25] 4/40 [10%];[21] 16/41 [36%];[22] 8/33 [24%];[23] 6/25 [24%][24]). One death was attributed to anorexia nervosa in the control group in one outpatient RCT with a 1 year follow up.[18] Three deaths attributed to anorexia nervosa occurred in the 5 year follow up period in one inpatient based RCT.[27]

Comment: All the RCTs were small and had limited power to detect clinically important differences if they existed. The amount of therapeutic input varied considerably between and within the RCTs. There was variation in methods of recruitment, reporting of key results (e.g. withdrawal rates), and the description of participants' characteristics and selection. The people in the inpatient RCTs covered a broad range of severity.[26]

| OPTION | ANTIDEPRESSANT MEDICATION |

Three small RCTs found no evidence of beneficial effects from the use of amitriptyline or fluoxetine.

Benefits: We found no systematic review. We found three small RCTs. The first RCT allocated 42 people with early onset and short duration anorexia nervosa (mean age 16.6 years, mean 27% below average weight, 1.5 years duration of anorexia nervosa) from two centres (5 outpatients) to amitriptyline or placebo.[28] Eighteen people refused to participate and two more in the amitriptyline group had low amitriptyline blood levels suggesting poor treatment adherence. The RCT found no difference between the groups on any outcome variable measured at 5 weeks. The second RCT (33 women; mean age 26.2 years; mean BMI (see glossary, p 8) 15.0 kg/m^2; mean duration of anorexia nervosa 8.0 years) compared fluoxetine 60 mg versus placebo for the duration (mean 36 days) of inpatient treatment (see glossary, p 8) (which included individual and group psychotherapy [see glossary, p 8]).[29] There were two early withdrawals from the fluoxetine group. The RCT found no significant differences in weight gain, eating symptoms, or depressive symptoms between the groups. The third RCT[30] compared amitriptyline, cyproheptadine, and placebo, and found no significant difference between treatments (see benefits under cyproheptadine, p 6).

Harms: None reported. General harms of tricyclic and other antidepressants are described in the section on depression (see depressive disorders, p 74). The QT interval may be prolonged in people with anorexia nervosa,[31] and tricyclic antidepressants (amitriptyline, protriptyline, nortriptyline, doxepin, maprotiline) also increase the QT interval.[32–34] In an observational study (495 people with mental illness and 101 healthy controls), an increased risk of QTc was seen with tricyclic use, adjusting for age and other drug use (adjusted OR 2.6, 95% CI 1.2 to 5.6).[35]

Comment: The RCTs were all of short duration. Prolongation of the QT interval may be associated with increased risk of ventricular tachycardia, torsades de pointes, and sudden death.[33,34]

OPTION	NEUROLEPTIC MEDICATION

We found no good evidence.

Benefits: We found no systematic review and no RCTs.

Harms: General harms of neuroleptics are described in the section on schizophrenia (see schizophrenia, p 127). The QT interval may be prolonged in people with anorexia nervosa,[31,32] and many neuroleptics (haloperidol, pimozide, sertindole, thioridazine, chlorpromazine, and others) may also increase the QT interval.[33,34] An observational study (495 people with mental illness and 101 healthy controls) found an increased risk of QTc with high and very high dose neuroleptic use after adjusting for age and other drug use (high dose: adjusted OR 3.4, 95% CI 1.2 to 10.1; very high dose: adjusted OR 5.6, 95% CI 1.6 to 19.3).[35]

Comment: Prolongation of the QT interval may be associated with increased risk of ventricular tachycardia, torsades de pointes, and sudden death.[33,34]

OPTION	ZINC

One RCT found no improvement in daily weight gain with the addition of zinc to an inpatient regime.

Benefits: We found no systematic review. We found one RCT (54 people aged > 15 years, mean BMI (see glossary, p 8) 15.8 kg/m^2, mean duration of anorexia nervosa 3.7 years, admitted to 2 eating disorder units), which compared 100 mg zinc gluconate versus placebo.[36] All but three of the people had normal zinc levels at pretreatment. Treatment was continued until the individual had gained 10% of weight over the admission weight on two consecutive weeks. Ten people in the zinc group and nine in the placebo group did not complete the study. There was no difference in average daily weight gain (zinc 0.079 kg v placebo 0.039 kg; difference 0.04 kg, 95% CI −0.005 to +0.08).

Harms: None reported.

Comment: None.

OPTION	CYPROHEPTADINE

One RCT in outpatients and two RCTs in inpatients found no significant difference between cyproheptadine and placebo in weight gain.

Benefits: We found no systematic review. We found three small RCTs. The first RCT (24 women in an outpatient setting) compared cyproheptadine versus placebo.[37] The trial found no significant difference in response to treatment after 2 months. The second RCT (81 women in 3 specialised inpatient centres) compared cyproheptadine versus placebo, and behaviour therapy versus no behaviour therapy.[38] The effect of behaviour therapy was not reported. There were no significant differences in weight gain between the cyproheptadine and placebo groups. The third RCT (72 women, mean age 20.6 years, mean 77% of target weight, mean duration of anorexia 2.9 years, at 2 specialised inpatient units) compared amitriptyline (up to a maximum of 160 mg) versus cyproheptadine (up to a maximum of 32 mg) versus placebo.[30] The drug treatment had no significant effect on treatment efficiency, i.e. the reciprocal of days to reach target weight times 90 (a dummy figure of 120 was used if people failed to reach target weight).

Harms: No harms were reported in the first two RCTs.[37,38] In the third RCT, on both day 7 and day 21, placebo exceeded the amitriptyline group in number of physical adverse events rated moderate or severe. Cyproheptadine had the lowest number of adverse effects. No one had to be withdrawn from the protocol because of adverse experiences.[30]

Comment: All three RCTs were of short duration.

OPTION	INPATIENT VERSUS OUTPATIENT TREATMENT SETTING IN ANOREXIA NERVOSA

We found weak evidence from one systematic review that outpatient treatment was as effective as inpatient treatment in those people not so severely ill as to warrant emergency intervention.

Benefits: We found one systematic review (search date 1999)[39] comparing inpatient (see glossary, p 8) with outpatient care. The review identified one RCT, which had a 5 year follow up.[40,41] Ninety people referred with anorexia nervosa (mean age 22 years, weight loss 26% of matched population mean weight, mean duration 3.2 years) were randomised to four treatment groups: inpatient treatment, outpatient treatment (individual and family therapy [see glossary, p 8]), outpatient group therapy, and assessment only. Assessors were not blind to treatment allocation. Adherence to allocated treatment (defined as accepting allocation and at least 1 attendance at a treatment group or individual treatment session) differed significantly between groups: inpatient treatment 18 of 30 (60%); outpatient treatment (individual and family therapy) 18 of 20 (90%); outpatient group psychotherapy (see glossary, p 8) 17 of 20 (85%); and assessment interview only 20 of 20 (100%). Treatment adherence differed significantly between outpatient and inpatient treatment (RR 1.46, 95% CI 1.06 to 2.0). Average acceptance of therapeutic input also varied between groups

(20 weeks inpatient treatment, 9 outpatient sessions, and 5 group sessions). In the assessment only group, six people had no treatment of any kind in the first year, and the others had treatment elsewhere (6 had inpatient treatment, 5 had outpatient hospital treatment, and 3 had at least weekly contact with their general practitioners). Six people in this group spent almost the entire year in treatment. There were no significant differences between any of the four groups at 1, 2, and 5 years mean weight or in the Morgan and Russell global scores (see glossary, p 8). The proportion of people with a good outcome with inpatient treatment was five of 29 (17%) at 2 years and nine of 27 (33%) at 5 years; with outpatient treatment (individual and family therapy) four of 20 (20%) at 2 years and eight of 17 (47%) at 5 years; with outpatient group psychotherapy five of 19 (26%) at 2 years and 10 of 19 (53%) at 5 years; and with assessment interview only two of 20 (10%) at 2 years and six of 19 (32%) at 5 years.

Harms: One person died as a result of anorexia nervosa between the assessment and the start of outpatient group treatment, and one of the people allocated to inpatient treatment died as a result of anorexia nervosa by 5 years.[40,41]

Comment: The systematic review[39] was unable to draw meaningful conclusions from numerous case series as participant characteristics, treatments, mortality, and outcomes varied widely. Individuals admitted for inpatient treatment had a lower mean weight than those treated as outpatients. One subsequent observational study (355 people with anorexia nervosa; 169 with anorexia nervosa bulimic type; mean age 25 years; mean duration of illness 5.7 years; 75% available for 2.5 years' follow up) found that people with longer duration of illness had a higher likelihood of good outcome with longer than with briefer duration of inpatient treatment, and those with a shorter duration of illness had a higher likelihood of good outcome with briefer inpatient treatment.[42] Median duration of inpatient treatment was 11.6 weeks for anorexia nervosa and 10.6 weeks for anorexia nervosa/bulimia nervosa.

OPTION   CISAPRIDE

One small RCT found no clear benefit from cisapride.

Benefits: We found no systematic review. We found one small RCT (34 inpatients aged 18–40 years at 2 hospitals; mean duration 2.7 years; BMI (see glossary, p 8) 15.1 kg/m^2) comparing cisapride (30 mg) versus placebo for 8 weeks.[43] The trial found no significant difference in weight gain (placebo 5.7 kg v cisapride 5.1 kg; P = NS).

Harms: No adverse events were noted in this RCT. The QT interval in anorexia nervosa is prolonged even in the absence of medication; therefore, cisapride is not recommended in anorexia nervosa. Cisapride has now been withdrawn in many countries because of an increased risk of cardiac irregularities, including ventricular tachycardia, torsades de pointes, and sudden death.[33,34]

Comment: Five people withdrew from the RCT and were not included in the analysis.

Anorexia nervosa

| QUESTION | What are the effects of interventions to prevent or treat complications of anorexia? |

| OPTION | HORMONAL TREATMENT |

We found no good evidence on the effects of hormonal treatment on fracture rates. One small RCT found no effect of oestrogen administration on bone mineral density.

Benefits: We found no systematic review. We found one RCT (48 women, mean age 23.7 years, mean duration of anorexia nervosa 4.0 years) of hormone replacement therapy (Premarin 0.625 mg on days 1–25 plus Provera 5 mg on days 16–25) versus an oral contraceptive containing 35 µg ethinyl oestradiol versus no medication.[44] All women maintained a calcium intake of 1500 mg using oral calcium carbonate. Spinal bone mineral density was measured at 6 monthly intervals. There was no significant difference in the final bone density at follow up of 0.5–3 years.

Harms: Three women withdrew from the oestrogen treatment; two because of adverse effects, and one woman withdrew from the control treatment.

Comment: Improvements in bone mineral density would not necessarily lead to reductions in risk of fractures.

GLOSSARY

Body mass index Weight (kg) divided by height (m) squared.

Dietary advice Dieticians with experience of eating disorders discuss diet, mood, and daily behaviours.

Family therapy Treatment that includes members of the family of origin or the constituted family, and that addresses the eating disorder as a problem of family life.

Inpatient treatment This has been regarded as the standard approach to the management of anorexia nervosa.[45] One of the key components of inpatient treatment is refeeding, which is achieved through structured, supervised meals. Psychotherapy (of a variety of different types) and pharmacotherapy are included in many programmes.

Morgan Russell scales A widely used measure of outcome for anorexia nervosa that consists of two scores: an average outcome score and a general outcome score. The average outcome score is based on the outcome in five areas: nutritional status, menstrual function, mental state, sexual adjustment, and socioeconomic status.

Psychotherapy Different types of psychological treatments given individually or in groups are included here. These use psychodynamic, cognitive behavioural, or supportive techniques, or combinations of these.

REFERENCES

1. American Psychiatric Association. *Diagnostic and Statistical Manual of Mental Disorders (DSM-IV)*. 4th ed. Washington DC: APA, 1994.

2. Pawluck DE, Gorey KM. Secular trends in the incidence of anorexia nervosa: integrative review of population-based studies. *Int J Eat Disord* 1998;23:347–352.

3. Råstam M, Gillberg C, Garton M. Anorexia nervosa in a Swedish urban region. A population-based study. *Br J Psychiatry* 1989;155:642–646.

4. Strober M, Freeman R, Lampert C, et al. Controlled family study of anorexia nervosa and bulimia nervosa: evidence of shared liability and transmission of partial syndromes. *Am J Psychiatry* 2000;157:393–401.

5. Lilenfeld LR, Kaye WH, Greeno CG, et al. A controlled family study of anorexia nervosa and bulimia nervosa: psychiatric disorders in first-degree relatives and effects of proband comorbidity. *Arch Gen Psychiatry* 1998;55:603–610.

6. Wade TD, Bulik CM, Neale M, et al. Anorexia nervosa and major depression: shared genetic and environmental risk factors. *Am J Psychiatry* 2000;157:469–471.

7. Fairburn CG, Cooper Z, Doll HA, Welch SL. Risk factors for anorexia nervosa: three integrated case-control comparisons. *Arch Gen Psychiatry* 1999;56:468–476.

8. Steinhausen, H-C. The course and outcome of anorexia nervosa. In: Brownell K, Fairburn CG, eds. *Eating Disorders and Obesity: a comprehensive handbook*. New York: The Guilford Press,1995:234–237.

9. Harri, EC, Barraclough B. Excess mortality of mental disorder. *Br J Psychiatry* 1998;173: 11–53.

10. Nielsen S, Møller-Madsen S, Isager T, Jørgensen J, Pagsberg K, Theander S. Standardized mortality in eating disorders: a quantitative summary of previously published and new evidence. *J Psychosom Res* 1998;44: 413–434.

11. Lucas A, Melton L, Crowson C, O'Fallon WM. Long term fracture risk among women with anorexia nervosa: a population-based cohort study. *Mayo Clin Proc* 1999;74:972–977.

12. Morgan HG, Russell GF. Value of family background and clinical features as predictors of long-term outcome in anorexia nervosa: four-year follow-up study of 41 patients. *Psychol Med* 1975;5:355–371.

13. Cooper Z, Fairburn CG. The Eating Disorders Examination. A semi-structured interview for the assessment of the specific psychopathology of eating disorders. *Int J Eat Disord* 1987;6:1–8.

14. Garner DM. *Eating Disorder Inventory-2 (EDI-2): professional manual*. Odessa FL: Psychological Assessment Resources Inc., 1991.

15. Garner DM, Garfinkel PE. The eating attitudes test: an index of the symptoms of anorexia nervosa. *Psychol Med* 1979;10:647–656.

16. Henderson M, Freeman CPL. A self-rating scale for bulimia: the 'BITE'. *Br J Psychiatry* 1987;150: 18–24.

17. Herzog T (in press). Stand der vergleichenden Therapieforschung bei Anorexia nervosa. Ergebnisse einer Systematischen Literaturübersicht. In: Gastpar M, Remschmidt HJ, Senf W, eds. *Forschungsperspektiven bei Esstorungen*. Berlin: Verlag Wissenschaft und Praxis.

18. Dare C, Eisler I, Russell G, Treasure J, Dodge L. Psychological therapies for adult patients with anorexia nervosa: a randomised controlled trial of outpatient treatments. *Br J Psychiatry* 2001;178: 216–221.

19. Hall A, Crisp AH. Brief psychotherapy in the treatment of anorexia nervosa. Outcome at one year. *Br J Psychiatry* 1987;151:185–191.

20. Serfaty MA. Cognitive therapy versus dietary counselling in the outpatient treatment of anorexia nervosa: effects of the treatment phase. *Eur Eat Dis Rev* 1999;7:334–350.

21. Eisler I, Dare C, Hodes M, Russell GFM, Dodge E, Le Grange D. Family therapy for adolescent anorexia nervosa: the results of a controlled comparison of two family interventions. *J Child Psychol Psychiatry* 2000;41: 727–736.

22. Robin AL, Siegel PT, Moye AW, et al. A controlled comparison of family versus individual therapy for adolescents with anorexia nervosa. *J Am Acad Child Adolesc Psychiatry* 1999;38:1482–1489.

23. Wallin U, Kronvall P, Majewski M-L. Body awareness therapy in teenage anorexia nervosa: outcome after 2 years. *Eur Eat Dis Rev* 2000;8: 19–30.

24. Geist R, Heinmaa M, Stephens D, et al. Comparison of family therapy and family group psychoeducation in adolescents with anorexia nervosa. *Can J Psychiatry* 2000;45: 173–178.

25. Treasure JL, Todd G, Brolly M, Tiller J, Nehmed A, Denman F. A pilot study of a randomized trial of cognitive analytical therapy vs educational behavioral therapy for adult anorexia nervosa. *Behav Res Ther* 1995;33:363–367.

26. Russell GFM, Szmukler G, Dare C, Eisler I. An evaluation of family therapy in anorexia nervosa and bulimia nervosa. *Arch Gen Psychiatry* 1987; 44:1047–1056.

27. Eisler I, Dare C, Russell GFM, Szmukler GI, Le Grange D, Dodge E. Family and individual therapy in anorexia nervosa. A 5-year follow-up. *Arch Gen Psychiatry* 1997;54:1025–1030.

28. Biederman J, Herzog DB, Rivinus TM, et al. Amitriptyline in the treatment of anorexia nervosa: a double-blind, placebo-controlled study. *J Clin Psychopharmacol* 1985;5:10–16.

29. Attia E, Haiman C, Walsh BT, et al. Does fluoxetine augment the inpatient treatment of anorexia nervosa? *Am J Psychiatry* 1998;155: 548–551.

30. Halmi KA, Eckert E, LaDu TJ, et al. Anorexia nervosa. Treatment efficacy of cyproheptadine and amitriptyline. *Arch Gen Psychiatry* 1986;43: 177–181.

31. Ackerman MJ. The long QT syndrome: ion channel diseases of the heart. *Mayo Clin Proc* 1998;73: 250–269.

32. Becker A, Grinspoon SK, Klibanski A, Herzog DB. Current concepts: eating disorders. *N Engl J Med* 1999;340:1092–1098.

33. Yap Y, Camm J. Risk of torsades de pointes with non-cardiac drugs: doctors need to be aware that many drugs can cause QT prolongation. *BMJ* 2000;320:1158–1159.

34. Sheridan DJ. Drug-induced proarrhythmic effects: assessment of changes in QT interval. *Br J Clin Pharm* 2000;50:297–302.

35. Reilly JG, Ayis SA, Ferrier IN, Jones SJ, Thomas SHL. QTc interval abnormalities and psychotropic drug therapy in psychiatric patients. *Lancet* 2000; 355:1048–1052.

36. Birmingham CL, Goldner EM, Bakan R. Controlled trial of zinc supplementation in anorexia nervosa. *Int J Eat Disord* 1994;15:251–255.

37. Vigersky RA, Loriaux L. The effect of cyproheptadine in anorexia nervosa: a double blind trial. In: Vigersky RA, ed. *Anorexia Nervosa*. New York: Raven Press,1977:349–356.

38. Goldberg SC, Halmi KA, Eckert RC, Casper RC, Davis JM. Cyproheptadine in anorexia nervosa. *Br J Psychiatry* 1979;134:67–70.

39. West Midlands Development and Evaluation Service. *In-patient Versus Out-patient Care for Eating Disorders*. DPHE 1999 Report No. 17. Birmingham: University of Birmingham, 1999. Search date 1999; primary sources Medline, Psychlit, Cochrane Library, variety of internet sites, and hand searches of relevant editions of relevant journals and references from identified articles.

40. Crisp AH, Norton K, Gowers S, et al. A controlled study of the effect of therapies aimed at adolescent and family psychopathology in anorexia nervosa. *Br J Psychiatry* 1991;159: 325–333.

41. Gowers S, Norton K, Halek C, Crisp AH. Outcome of outpatient psychotherapy in a random allocation treatment study of anorexia nervosa. *Int J Eat Disord* 1994;15:65–177.

42. Kächele H for the study group MZ-ESS. Eine multizentrische Studie zu Aufwand und Erfolg bei psychodynamischer Therapie von Eβstörungen. *Psychother Med Psychol (Stuttg)* 1999;49: 100–108.

43. Szmukler GI, Young GP, Miller G, et al. A controlled trial of cisapride in anorexia nervosa. *Int J Eat Disord* 1995;17:347–357.

44. Klibanski A, Biller BMK, Schoenfeld DA, Herzog DB, Saxe VC. The effects of estrogen administration on trabecular bone loss in young women with anorexia nervosa. *J Clin Endocrinol Metab* 1995;80:898–904.

45. American Psychiatric Association. Practice guideline for the treatment of patients with eating disorders (revision). *Am J Psychiatry* 157:1(suppl):1–39.

Janet Treasure
Psychiatrist
Institute of Psychiatry Kings College
London
London
UK

Ulrike Schmidt
Psychiatrist
South London and Maudsley NHS Trust
London
UK

Competing interests: None declared.

Attention deficit hyperactivity disorder in children

Search date June 2001

Paul Ramchandani, Carol Joughin and Morris Zwi

QUESTIONS

Effects of treatments for attention deficit hyperactivity disorder in children 13

INTERVENTIONS

Likely to be beneficial
Methylphenidate 13
Dexamfetamine 15
Methylphenidate plus behavioural treatment 17

Unknown effectiveness
Clonidine 15
Psychological/behavioural treatment 16

See glossary, p 18

Key Messages

- One systematic review has found that methylphenidate versus placebo reduces core symptoms of attention deficit hyperactivity disorder in the short term but may disturb sleep and appetite. The review could not draw firm conclusions about the effects of methylphenidate versus dexamfetamine or tricyclic antidepressants. The review also found that methylphenidate versus psychological/behavioural treatment improves symptoms in the medium term, but the clinical importance of these findings is unclear.

- Limited evidence from two systematic reviews suggests that dexamfetamine versus placebo improves some behavioural outcomes but the clinical importance of these findings is unclear.

- Limited evidence from one systematic review suggests that clonidine versus placebo reduces core attention deficit hyperactivity disorder symptoms, but the clinical importance of these findings is unclear.

- One systematic review of two small RCTs found insufficient evidence about psychological or behavioural treatments; one subsequent RCT found no significant difference between psychological/behavioural treatment versus standard care in behavioural rating scales.

- One systematic review found inconsistent results for combination treatments (medication plus psychological/behavioural treatment) versus placebo in attention deficit hyperactivity disorder. A second systematic review has found that combination treatments versus psychological/behavioural treatments alone significantly improve attention deficit hyperactivity disorder symptoms.

Attention deficit hyperactivity disorder in children

DEFINITION   Attention deficit hyperactivity disorder is "a persistent pattern of inattention and/or hyperactivity and impulsivity that is more frequent and severe than is typically observed in individuals at a comparable level of development" (DSM-IV).[1] Inattention, hyperactivity, and impulsivity are commonly known as the core symptoms of attention deficit hyperactivity disorder. Symptoms must be present for at least 6 months, observed before the age of 7 years, and "clinically significant impairment in social, academic, or occupational functioning" must be evident in more than one setting. The symptoms must not be better explained by another disorder such as an anxiety disorder (see glossary, p 18), mood disorder, psychosis, or autistic disorder.[1] The World Health Organization's International Statistical Classification of Diseases and Related Health Problems (ICD-10)[2] uses the term "hyperkinetic disorder" for a more restricted diagnosis. It differs from the DSM-IV classification[3] as all three problems of attention, hyperactivity, and impulsiveness must be present, more stringent criteria for "pervasiveness" across situations must be met, and the presence of another disorder is an exclusion criterion.

INCIDENCE/ PREVALENCE   Prevalence estimates of attention deficit hyperactivity disorder vary according to the diagnostic criteria used and the population sampled. DSM-IV prevalence estimates among school children range from 3–5%,[1] but other estimates vary from 1.7–16%.[4,5] No objective test exists to confirm the diagnosis of attention deficit hyperactivity disorder, which remains a clinical diagnosis. Other conditions frequently coexist with attention deficit hyperactivity disorder. Oppositional defiant disorder (see glossary, p 18) is present in 35% (95% CI 27% to 44%) of children with attention deficit hyperactivity disorder, conduct disorder (see glossary, p 18) in 26% (95% CI 13% to 41%), anxiety disorder in 26% (95% CI 18% to 35%), and depressive disorder (see glossary, p 18) in 18% (95% CI 11% to 27%).[6]

AETIOLOGY/ RISK FACTORS   The underlying causes of attention deficit hyperactivity disorder are not known.[6] There is limited evidence that it has a genetic component.[7–9] Risk factors also include psychosocial factors.[10] There is increased risk in boys compared to girls, with ratios varying from 3:1[6] to 4:1.[3]

PROGNOSIS   More than 70% of hyperactive children may continue to meet criteria for attention deficit hyperactivity disorder in adolescence, and up to 65% of adolescents may continue to meet criteria for attention deficit hyperactivity disorder in adulthood.[5] Changes in diagnostic criteria cause difficulty with interpretation of the few outcome studies. One cohort of boys followed up for an average of 16 years found a ninefold increase in antisocial personality disorder and a fourfold increase in substance misuse disorder.[7]

AIMS   To reduce inattention, hyperactivity and impulsivity, and to improve psychosocial and educational functioning in affected children and adolescents, with minimal adverse effects of treatment.

OUTCOMES   Children's behaviour, such as Conners Teacher's Rating Scales (see glossary, p 18); school performance, such as School Situations Questionnaire (see glossary, p 18); adverse effects.

METHODS   *Clinical Evidence* search and appraisal June 2001.

| OPTION | METHYLPHENIDATE |

One systematic review has found that methylphenidate versus placebo reduces core symptoms of attention deficit hyperactivity disorder in the short term but may disturb sleep and appetite. The review could not draw firm conclusions about the effects of methylphenidate versus dexamfetamine or tricyclic antidepressants. The review also found that methylphenidate versus psychological/behavioural treatment improves symptoms in the medium term, but the clinical importance of these findings is unclear.

Benefits: We found one systematic review (search date 2000).[11] Most studies were conducted in the USA, used a diagnosis of attention deficit disorder (DSM-III) or attention deficit hyperactivity disorder (DSM-IIIR or DSM-IV), and included children aged between 5–18 years, mostly recruited from psychiatric and other hospital out-patient clinics. **Versus placebo:** The systematic review included, but did not pool results from, 13 rigorously selected short term RCTs (1177 children, aged 5–18 years).[11] Three RCTs (99 children) found no significant difference in core symptoms between methylphenidate versus placebo. The other 10 RCTs found that methylphenidate (dose range 0.56–0.72 mg/kg daily or 5–35 mg daily for trials reporting in those units) versus placebo significantly improved the Conners Teacher's Rating Scale (see glossary, p 18) hyperactivity index (see comment below). The same systematic review found similar results in 17 other RCTs (643 children), which were less stringent in terms of homogeneity of participants, outcome measures, and methodological quality. **Versus dexamfetamine:** The systematic review[11] identified four poorly reported crossover RCTs (224 children, aged 5–18 years) comparing methylphenidate (dose range 0.6 mg–4.5 mg/kg daily or 20 mg daily for trials reporting in those units) versus dexamfetamine (dose 0.39–2.6 mg/kg daily or 10 mg daily for trials reporting in those units) but, because of heterogeneity, could not pool their results. Three RCTs (99 children, aged 5–12 years) found no significant difference with methylphenidate versus dexamfetamine in the outcomes of interest. The other RCT found improvement with methylphenidate versus dexamfetamine for some, but not all outcome measures. No firm conclusions can be drawn. **Versus tricyclic antidepressants:** The systematic review[11] identified, but could not pool, the results of two poorly reported crossover RCTs (105 children) comparing methylphenidate (dose 0.4 mg/kg daily or mean 20 mg daily for trials reporting in those units) versus imipramine (dose 1–2 mg/kg daily or mean 65 mg daily for trials reporting in those units). One RCT (75 children) found no significant differences in clinical outcomes after 1 year, and the other RCT (30 children) found that imipramine versus methylphenidate improved some but not all outcomes in the short term. No firm conclusions can be drawn. **Versus psychological/behavioural treatment:** We found one systematic review (search date 2000) that identified four RCTs comparing methylphenidate versus psychological/behavioural

Attention deficit hyperactivity disorder in children

treatment (see glossary, p 18).[11] Three of the RCTs (192 children, aged 5–12 years) were poorly reported and compared a variety of psychological/behavioural treatments (individual cognitive training [see glossary, p 18] over 12 wks; parent and teacher training; behaviour treatment for 8 wks) versus methylphenidate (5–60 mg daily). Overall, these three RCTs found limited evidence that, in the medium term, methylphenidate versus psychological/behavioural treatment improved symptoms. The fourth RCT (579 children, aged 7–10 years) compared medication treatment (144 children, double blind titration of methylphenidate dose, switched to alternative medication after 28 days if response unsatisfactory, mean initial dose 30.5 mg daily) versus intensive behavioural management versus combined medication and intensive behavioural management versus standard community care.[12] A total of 74% of the children in the medication group were taking methylphenidate at the end of the study. Initial results were not presented as the number of children who improved, but only as P values. Methylphenidate versus psychological/behaviour treatment improved some, but not all, of the symptoms of attention deficit disorder. Subsequent secondary analysis has developed these findings (see comment below).

Harms: The systematic review (search date 2000)[11] did not combine results on harms because of heterogeneity and incomplete data reporting. It presented the number of RCTs that had found significant results (see comment below). **Versus placebo:** The following symptoms were found by at least one RCT to be significantly more common in children receiving methylphenidate: sleep disorders; anorexia or appetite disturbance; headache; motor tics; irritability; and abdominal pain (see table 1, p 20). We found no good evidence of effects of methylphenidate on growth rates in children. **Versus dexamfetamine:** Out of the four RCTs identified by the systematic review, two RCTs reported no significant difference with methylphenidate versus dexamfetamine for anorexia or appetite disturbance and one RCT reported no significant difference in motor tics, abdominal pain, and irritability. **Versus psychological/ behavioural treatment:** The one large RCT comparing medication with intensive behavioural treatment (see glossary, p 18)[12] found that, of the children receiving either medication management or combined medication and intensive behavioural treatment, 50% reported mild adverse effects, 11% had moderate adverse effects, and 3% experienced severe adverse effects.

Comment: The RCT comparing medication versus intensive behavioural treatment is the largest and most rigorous currently available RCT of attention deficit hyperactivity disorder treatments.[12] Subsequent secondary analysis suggests that 56% of the children taking medication improved compared to 34% of these in the behavioural treatment group.[13] There is also a suggestion that children with comorbid behaviour problems (oppositional defiant disorder/ conduct disorder) demonstrated a stronger response to medication than those without comorbid behaviour problems, and that children with attention deficit hyperactivity disorder and anxiety disorders were likely to respond equally well to behavioural or medication treatments.[14] There are some concerns about the methods used in the RCT and caution should be exercised when using the results of secondary analysis, as they are more susceptible to bias than the primary outcome analyses.[15] It should also be noted that the principal outcome measures were rating scales based on impressions of parents and teachers; they did not include the child's view or direct measures of their response to treatment. Long term effects on psychosocial adjustment, educational success, or behavioural improvement are unclear. We found no evidence about methylphenidate for pre-school children.[16] The abbreviated Conners Teacher's Rating Scale has been used widely in treatment studies and has been researched, validated, and standardised to measure treatment effects in attention deficit hyperactivity disorder.[17] However, the clinical importance of the effect of methylphenidate versus placebo on the abbreviated Conners Teacher's Rating Scale remains unclear.

OPTION   DEXAMFETAMINE SULPHATE

Limited evidence from two systematic reviews suggests that dexamfetamine versus placebo improved some behavioural outcomes but the clinical importance of these findings is unclear.

Benefits: **Versus placebo:** We found two systematic reviews.[5,16] The first systematic review (search date 1997, 4 RCTs, 61 children aged 6–12 years, dexamfetamine 0.46–0.75 mg/kg daily) found that dexamfetamine versus placebo improved the change in the abbreviated Conners Teacher's Rating Scale (see glossary, p 18) (WMD −4.8, 95% CI −6.4 to −2.9).[16] The second later systematic review (search date 1997, 3 RCTs, 150 children aged 6–16 years, dexamfetamine 5–20 mg daily) only evaluated longer term studies (> 12 wks).[5] It found some evidence of positive outcomes (including improved concentration and hyperactivity) with dexamfetamine versus placebo. However, some methodological problems were identified with the studies in this review.[5] The clinical importance of these findings is unclear. **Versus methylphenidate:** See benefits of methylphenidate, p 13.

Harms: **Versus placebo:** The second systematic review found that dexamfetamine significantly increased anorexia and appetite disturbance in three RCTs.[5] **Versus methylphenidate:** See harms of methylphenidate, p 14.

Comment: See comment of methylphenidate for the principal outcome measures, p 14.

OPTION   CLONIDINE

Limited evidence from one systematic review suggests that clonidine versus placebo reduced core attention deficit hyperactivity disorder symptoms, but the clinical importance of these findings is unclear.

Benefits: **Versus placebo:** We found one systematic review (search date 1999, 6 RCTs, 143 children, mean age 11 years, dose of clonidine 0.1–0.24 mg daily for 4–12 wks).[18] One of the six RCTs was a comparison of clonidine versus methylphenidate, rather than versus placebo,[19] and the rating scales of the clinical features of attention deficit hyperactivity disorder completed by parents, teachers, and clinicians were combined in the systematic review. A meta-analysis of the six RCTs found that clonidine versus placebo improved this combined rating scale (effect size 0.58, 95% CI 0.27 to 0.89). The clinical importance of this result is unclear (see comment below), and the results should be treated with caution. **Versus methylphenidate or combined treatment:** We found no systematic review but found one small RCT (3 groups of 8 boys aged 6–16 years with attention deficit hyperactivity disorder and either comorbid oppositional defiant disorder [see glossary, p 18] or conduct disorder [see glossary, p 18]) comparing clonidine (mean dose 0.17 mg daily) versus methylphenidate (mean dose 35 mg daily) versus clonidine plus methylphenidate.[19] Most outcomes were not significantly different between the three groups. However, methylphenidate versus clonidine significantly improved the teacher reported School Situations Questionnaire (see glossary, p 18) (P < 0.009). The clinical importance of this isolated result from a single small RCT is unclear.

Harms: **Versus placebo:** The systematic review[18] included information from 10 studies of harms. Not all were high quality RCTs, and their results are difficult to interpret. In children taking clonidine, nine of 10 studies found sedation in children; six studies found increased irritability. Electrocardiographs were recorded in two placebo controlled RCTs, which found no abnormalities. **Versus methylphenidate or combined treatment:** One small RCT (24 boys)[19] found that two of eight children on clonidine developed new onset bradycardia. Four of eight children on a combination of clonidine and methylphenidate developed bradycardia.

Comment: The systematic review[18] noted larger effect sizes in smaller and lower quality studies. Inclusion of the RCT of clonidine versus methylphenidate[19] in the systematic review creates difficulties in using that review to indicate the effects of clonidine versus placebo. The RCT[19] had a larger effect size than most other included studies, and it is likely to have inflated the final result of the meta-analysis. The results used by the systematic review for that RCT were not described in the original RCT report, and may have been a less reliable comparison of baseline and end of the study measures rather than a rigorous comparison of randomly allocated groups. Harms were reported as the number of studies that recorded a specific adverse effect or not rather then the number of children experiencing adverse effects.

OPTION	PSYCHOLOGICAL/BEHAVIOURAL TREATMENT

One systematic review of two small RCTs found insufficient evidence; one subsequent RCT found no significant difference with psychological/ behavioural treatment versus standard care in behavioural rating scales.

Benefits: **Versus standard care:** We found one systematic review (search date 1997, 2 RCTs, 50 children aged 6–13 years),[16] and a subsequent RCT.[12] The systematic review found no significant difference between psychological/behavioural treatment (see glossary, p 18) versus standard care in teacher rating scales (SMD −0.40, 95% CI −1.28 to +0.48) or parent ratings (1 RCT, 26 children, WMD −3.8, CI −9.6 to +2.0). The RCTs identified by the systematic review were small and the clinical importance of these results is unclear. The subsequent RCT (290 children)[12] found no significant difference between intensive behavioural treatments versus standard community care. In children with comorbid anxiety disorders (see glossary, p 18), the RCT found that intensive behavioural treatment resulted in better clinical outcomes. **Versus methylphenidate:** See benefits of methylphenidate, p 13.

Harms: Harms were not reported.

Comment: Children in the trials had different diagnoses, presentations, and clinical needs. Secondary analysis of one RCT[12] suggests small benefit with intensive behavioural treatment versus standard community care (34% of children improved with intensive behavioural treatment v 25% with standard community care group).[13] However, caution should be exercised in interpreting the results of secondary analysis as they are more susceptible to bias than the primary outcome analyses.[15]

OPTION   **MEDICATION PLUS PSYCHOLOGICAL/BEHAVIOURAL TREATMENT**

One systematic review found inconsistent results for combination treatments (medication plus psychological/behavioural treatment) versus placebo in attention deficit hyperactivity disorder. A second systematic review has found that combination treatments versus psychological/behavioural treatments alone significantly improve attention deficit hyperactivity disorder symptoms.

Benefits: **Versus control/placebo:** We found one systematic review (search date 1997, 3 RCTs, 35 children aged 5–13 years).[16] It found that combination of medication with psychological/behavioural treatments versus control/placebo improved parent ratings of attention deficit hyperactivity disorder (Conners Parent's Rating Scale WMD −7.3, 95% CI −12.3 to −2.4), but not teacher ratings of attention deficit hyperactivity disorder (Conners Teacher's Rating Scale [see glossary, p 18] WMD 1.3, 95% CI −0.7 to +3.2). The clinical importance of these findings is unclear.[16] **Versus stimulant drugs alone:** See benefits of methylphenidate, p 13. **Versus psychological/behavioural treatments alone:** We found one systematic review (search date 2000, 11 RCTs, 428 children aged 5–18 years).[11] It found that methylphenidate plus behavioural treatments versus behavioural treatments alone significantly improved attention deficit hyperactivity disorder behaviours, symptoms, and measures of academic achievement. No significant difference was found in social skills or in measures of the relationship between parents and children.[11] The review separately assessed one RCT,[12] which found that combined drug and intensive behavioural treatment versus intensive behavioural treatment alone significantly improved three of five measures of attention deficit hyperactivity disorder core symptoms (see glossary, p 18), one of three measures of aggression/oppositional behaviour, one of three measures of anxiety depression, and one of three measures of academic achievement.[12]

Harms: The RCTs found no evidence of adverse effects. See harms of methylphenidate, p 14.

Comment: The RCT[12] is the largest and most methodologically rigorous study of attention deficit hyperactivity disorder treatments with high standards for reporting and follow up of nearly all children (see comment under methylphenidate, p 14).[15] The results of a secondary analysis of this RCT[12] suggest that children with attention deficit hyperactivity disorder and comorbid anxiety respond equally well to medication management or intensive behavioural treatment (see comment of methylphenidate about secondary analysis, p 14);[14] however, secondary analysis indicated that combined medication management plus intensive behavioural treatment was better than medication management alone.[14]

GLOSSARY

Anxiety disorder A range of conditions with features including apprehension, motor tension, and autonomic overactivity.

Behavioural treatment Treatment using insights from learning theory to achieve specific changes in behaviour. It is usually highly structured. It can be used with either children with attention deficit hyperactivity disorder or their parents/carers.

Cognitive training Brief structured treatment aimed at changing dysfunctional beliefs.

Conduct disorder Conduct disorders include a repetitive pattern of antisocial, aggressive, or defiant conduct, which violate age appropriate social expectations.[2]

Conners Teacher's Rating Scales Widely used rating scales for assessment of symptoms of attention deficit hyperactivity disorder used extensively in both clinical work and epidemiological studies. There are 10 item parent and teacher questionnaires which can be used for children aged 3–17 years.

Core symptoms Inattention, hyperactivity, and impulsivity are commonly known as the core symptoms of attention deficit hyperactivity disorder.[5]

Depressive disorder Characterised by persistent low mood, loss of interest and enjoyment, and reduced energy.

Oppositional defiant disorder The presence of markedly defiant, disobedient, provocative behaviour, but without the severely dissocial or aggressive acts seen in conduct disorder.[2]

Psychological/behavioural treatments Includes any of the following methods: contingency management methods (e.g. behaviour modification); cognitive–behavioural therapy; individual psychotherapy; parent training or education; teacher training and education; parent and family counselling/therapy; social skills training; and electroencephalogram, biofeedback, or relaxation treatment.

School Situations Questionnaire A teacher completed questionnaire, which measures the pervasiveness of child behaviour problems across 12 school situations.[20]

REFERENCES

1. American Psychiatric Association. *Diagnostic and Statistical Manual of Mental Disorders, 4th Edition (DSM-IV)*. American Psychiatric Association, Washington DC, 1994.

2. World Health Organization. *International Statistical Classification of Diseases and Related Health Problems, Tenth Revision, Vol 3*. Geneva; World Health Organization, 1994.

3. Taylor E, Sergeant J, Doepfner M, et al. Clinical guidelines for hyperkinetic disorder. European Society for Child and Adolescent Psychiatry. *Eur Child Adolesc Psychiatry* 1998;7:184–200.

4. Goldman LS, Genel M, Bezman RJ, Slanetz PJ. Diagnosis and treatment of attention-deficit/hyperactivity disorder in children and adolescents. Council on Scientific Affairs, American Medical Association. *JAMA* 1998;279:1100–1107.

5. Jadad AR, Boyle M, Cunningham C, Kim M, Schachar R. *Treatment of attention-deficit/hyperactivity disorder*. Evidence report/technology assessment: No 11 (Prepared by McMaster University under Contract No. 290–97-0017). Rockville MD, 1999. Agency for Health Care Policy and Research and Quality. Search date 1997; primary sources Medline, Cinahl, HealthStar,

PsychInfo, Embase, Cochrane Library, hand searched reference lists, and organisations funding research on attention deficit hyperactivity disorder and researchers contacted. http://hstat.nlm.nih.gov/hq.Hquest/screen/DirectAccess/db/3143.

6. Green M, Wong M, Atkins D, et al. *Diagnosis and treatment of attention-deficit/hyperactivity disorder in children and adolescents.* Council on Scientific Affairs, American Medical Association. Technical Review No.3 (Prepared by Technical Resources International, Inc. under Contract No. 290-94-2024.). Agency for Health Care Policy and Research, AHCPR Publication No. 99-0050. Rockville MD, 1999.

7. Finkel MF. The diagnosis and treatment of the adult attention deficit hyperactivity disorders. *Neurologist* 1997;3:31–44.

8. Hertzig MEE, Farber EAE. *Annual progress in child psychiatry and child development, 1996.* New York: Brunner/Mazel Inc, 1997:602.

9. Kaminester DD. Attention deficit hyperactivity disorder and methylphenidate: When society misunderstands medicine. *McGill J Med* 1997;3:105–114.

10. Taylor E, Sandberg S, Thorley G, Giles S. *The epidemiology of childhood hyperactivity.* London, Institute of Psychiatry. Maudsley Monographs 1991;33.

11. Lord J, Paisley S. *The clinical effectiveness and cost-effectiveness of methylphenidate for hyperactivity in childhood.* London: National Institute for Clinical Excellence, Version 2, August 2000. Search date 2000; primary sources Jadad et al. (reference 5 above), Medline, Cinahl, Healthstar, PsychInfo, and Embase.

12. Jensen PS, Arnold LE, Richters JE, et al. A 14-month randomized clinical trial of treatment strategies for attention-deficit/hyperactivity disorder. The MTA Cooperative Group. Multimodal Treatment Study of Children with ADHD. *Arch Gen Psychiatry* 1999;56:1073–1086.

13. Swanson JM, Kraemer HC, Hinshaw SP, et al. Clinical relevance of the primary findings of the MTA; success rates based on severity of ADHD and ODD symptoms at the end of treatment. *J Am Acad Child Adolesc Psychiatry* 2001;40:168–179.

14. Jensen PS, Hinshaw SP, Kraemer HP, Lenora N, et al. ADHD comorbidity findings from MTA study: comparing comorbid subgroups. *J Am Acad Child Adolesc Psychiatry* 2001;40:147–158.

15. Boyle MH, Jadad AR. Lessons from large trials: the MTA study as a model for evaluating the treatment of childhood psychiatric disorder. *Can J Psychiatry* 1999;44:991–998.

16. Miller A, Lee SK, Raina P, Klassen A, Zupanic J, Olsen L. A review of therapies for attention-deficit/hyperactivity disorder. 1998. Canadian Coordinating Office for Health Technology Assessment. Search date 1997; primary sources Medline, Current Contents, hand search of review articles, textbooks, British Columbia Methylphenidate Survey, and Intercontinental Medical Statistics for information on drug prescription and utilization in Canada.

17. Goyette CH, Conners CK, Ulrich RF. Normative data on revised Conners parent and teacher rating scales. *J Abnorm Child Psychol* 1978;6:221–236.

18. Connor DF, Fletcher KE, Swanson JM. A meta-analysis of clonidine for symptoms of attention-deficit hyperactivity disorder. *J Am Acad Child Adolesc Psychiatry* 1999;38:1551–1559. Search date 1999; primary sources Medline, PsychInfo, Current Contents, Social and Behavioral Sciences, and Current Contents Clinical Medicine, and hand searches of non-peer reviewed research reports, book chapters, chapter bibliographies, and individual report references.

19. Connor DF, Barkley RA, Davis HT. A pilot study of methylphenidate, clonidine, or the combination in ADHD comorbid with aggressive oppositional defiant or conduct disorder. *Clin Pediatr (Phila)* 2000;39:15–25.

20. Barkley RA. *Attention-Deficit Hyperactivity Disorder: A handbook for diagnosis and treatment.* New York: Guilford Press, 1990.

Paul Ramchandani
MRC Research Training Fellow, University of Oxford
Department of Psychiatry, Warneford Hospital, Oxford, UK

Carol Joughin
Project Manager
FOCUS Royal College of Psychiatrists Research Unit, London, UK

Morris Zwi
Consultant Child and Adolescent Psychiatrist
Child and Family Consultation Centre, Richmond, Surrey, UK

Competing interests: None declared. The opinions expressed are those of the authors and do not necessarily reflect those of the Royal College of Psychiatrists.

TABLE 1	The number of RCTs reporting significant adverse effects with methylphenidate versus placebo (see text, p 14).[11]

Adverse effect	Number of trials
Anorexia or appetite disturbance	7/12 (58%)
Motor tics	1/2 (50%)
Irritability	2/9 (22%)
Sleep disorder	4/20 (20%)
Abdominal pain	2/10 (20%)
Headache	2/10 (20%)

INTERVENTIONS

Key Messages

Psychotherapy

- Systematic reviews have found that cognitive behavioural therapy versus remaining on a waiting list reduces specific symptoms of bulimia nervosa, and improves non-specific symptoms such as depression.

- One systematic review and one subsequent RCT have found that non-cognitive psychotherapies versus waiting list controls improve the symptoms of bulimia nervosa.

- One well designed RCT found that cognitive behavioural therapy was more effective than interpersonal psychotherapy at 20 weeks, but the difference was not maintained 4 months later.

Antidepressants

- Systematic reviews have found that antidepressants reduce bulimic symptoms in the short term, but we found insufficient evidence about their role in maintenance treatment.

- We found insufficient evidence about the effects of different classes of antidepressants.

- One systematic review comparing antidepressants with psychotherapy found no significant difference in bulimic symptoms.

Combinations of antidepressants and psychotherapy

- One systematic review has found that combination treatment (antidepressants plus psychotherapy) versus antidepressants alone reduces binge frequency and depressive symptoms but not binge eating remission rates. It also found that combination treatment versus psychotherapy alone reduced short term remission from binge eating and depressive symptoms but had no significant effect on binge eating frequency.

DEFINITION   Bulimia nervosa (see glossary, p 29) is an intense preoccupation with body weight and shape, with regular episodes of uncontrolled overeating of large amounts of food (binge eating — see glossary, p 29) associated with use of extreme methods to counteract the feared effects of overeating. If a person also meets the diagnostic criteria for anorexia nervosa, then the diagnosis of anorexia nervosa takes precedence.[1] Bulimia nervosa can be difficult to identify because of extreme secrecy about binge eating and purgative behaviour. Weight may be normal but there is often a history of anorexia nervosa or restrictive dieting. Some people alternate between anorexia nervosa and bulimia nervosa.

INCIDENCE/   In community based studies, the prevalence of bulimia nervosa is
PREVALENCE between 0.5% and 1.0% in young women, with an even social class distribution.[2–4] About 90% of people diagnosed with bulimia nervosa are women. The numbers presenting with bulimia nervosa in industrialised countries increased during the decade that followed its recognition in the late 1970s and "a cohort effect" is reported in community surveys,[2,5,6] implying an increase in incidence. The prevalence of eating disorders such as bulimia nervosa is lower in non-industrialised populations,[7] and varies across ethnic groups. African-American women have a lower rate of restrictive dieting than white American women, but have a similar rate of recurrent binge eating.[8]

AETIOLOGY/   Young women from the developed world who restrict their dietary
RISK FACTORS intake are at greatest risk of developing bulimia nervosa and other eating disorders. One community based case control study compared 102 people with bulimia nervosa with 204 healthy controls and found higher rates of the following in people with the eating disorder: obesity, mood disorder, sexual and physical abuse, parental obesity, substance misuse, low self esteem, perfectionism, disturbed family dynamics, parental weight/shape concern, and early menarche.[9] Compared with a control group of 102 women who had other psychiatric disorders, women with bulimia nervosa had higher rates of parental problems and obesity.

PROGNOSIS   A 10 year follow up study (50 people with bulimia nervosa from a former trial of mianserin treatment) found that 52% had fully recovered, and only 9% continued to experience symptoms of bulimia nervosa.[10] A larger study (222 people from a trial of antidepressants and structured intensive group psychotherapy) found that, after a mean follow up of 11.5 years, 11% still met criteria for bulimia nervosa, whereas 70% were in full or partial remission.[11] Short term studies found similar results: about 50% of people made a full recovery, 30% made a partial recovery, and 20% continued to be symptomatic.[12] There are few consistent predictors of longer term outcome. Good prognosis has been associated with shorter illness duration, a younger age of onset, higher social class, and a family history of alcoholism.[10] Poor prognosis has been associated with a history of substance misuse,[11] premorbid and paternal obesity,[13] and, in some studies, personality disorder.[14–17] One study (102 people) of the natural course of bulimia nervosa found that 31% still had the disorder at 15 months and 15% at 5 years.[18] Only 28% received treatment during the follow up period. In an evaluation of response to cognitive behavioural therapy (see glossary, p 29), early progress (by session six) best predicted outcome.[19] A subsequent systematic review of the outcome literature found no consistent evidence to support early intervention and a better prognosis.[20]

AIMS To reduce symptoms of bulimia nervosa; to improve general psychiatric symptoms; to improve social functioning and quality of life.

OUTCOMES Frequency of binge eating, abstinence from binge eating, frequency of behaviours to reduce weight and counter the effects of binge eating, severity of extreme weight and shape preoccupation, severity of general psychiatric symptoms, severity of depression, improvement in social and adaptive functioning, remission rates, relapse rates, and withdrawal rates.

METHODS *Clinical Evidence* search and appraisal September 2001 and hand-search of reference lists from identified reviews. One systematic review was not included because it included uncontrolled studies.[21]

QUESTION **What are the effects of treatments for bulimia nervosa in adults?**

OPTION **COGNITIVE BEHAVIOURAL THERAPY**

Systematic reviews have found that cognitive behavioural therapy versus remaining on a waiting list reduces specific symptoms of bulimia nervosa and improves non-specific symptoms such as depression. One RCT has found that cognitive behavioural therapy versus interpersonal psychotherapy significantly reduces binge eating in the short term, but there was no significant difference in the long term. One subsequent RCT found significantly higher abstinence rates for subjects receiving cognitive behavioural therapy versus those in a support group.

Benefits: We found three systematic reviews of psychotherapy,[22–24] three subsequent RCTs,[25–27] and two subsequent analyses.[28,29] The third systematic review is in German and may be included in a future *Clinical Evidence* update.[25] The first systematic review (search date 2000, 27 RCTs) included RCTs of other binge eating disorders (see glossary, p 29), although most studies were of people with bulimia nervosa (see glossary, p 29) (18 RCTs in people with bulimia nervosa characterised by purging behaviour).[22] The second review (search date 1998, 26 RCTs) used a broad definition of cognitive behavioural therapy (CBT) (see glossary, p 29), including exposure and response prevention, and included non-randomised trials.[23] **Versus waiting list controls:** The first review (individual analyses included a maximum of 10 RCTs and 668 people) found that CBT versus remaining on a waiting list increased the proportion of people abstaining from binge eating at the end of the trial (7 RCTs; RR 0.64, 95% CI 0.53 to 0.78) and reduced depression scores (4 RCTs, 159 people) (see table 1, p 32).[22] Weight at the end of treatment was similar with CBT and remaining on the waiting list (3 RCTs). The review found insufficient evidence about other outcomes such as social functioning. The second systematic review (9 RCTs of specific CBT, 173 people) found that abstinence from binge eating at the end of treatment ranged from 33% to 92% (mean 55%).[23]

Pooled effect sizes (weighted for sample size) ranged from 1.22–1.35 for reduction in binge eating frequency, purging frequency, depression, and disturbed eating attitudes. Tests for heterogeneity were not significant. In one of the included RCTs, the benefits of CBT were maintained for up to 5 years.[13] **Versus placebo medication:** One subsequent RCT (91 people) found no significant difference in efficacy with unguided manual based self help CBT versus placebo medication (see benefits of antidepressants, p 26).[27] **Versus other psychotherapies:** The first review found that more people abstained from binge eating after CBT than after other psychotherapies, but the difference did not quite reach significance (7 RCTs; RR 0.80, 95% CI 0.61 to 1.04).[23] CBT in a full or less intensive form was not significantly superior to CBT in a pure self help form (see glossary, p 30) (4 RCTs; RR 0.90, 95% CI 0.74 to 1.10). CBT was associated with significantly lower depression scores at the end of treatment compared with other psychotherapies (8 RCTs, 273 people; SMD –0.52, 95% CI –0.76 to –0.27). CBT plus exposure therapy was not significantly more effective than CBT alone (3 RCTs; RR for abstinence from binge eating 0.87, 95% CI 0.65 to 1.16). Depression scores were significantly lower at the end of treatment with CBT plus exposure therapy versus CBT alone (3 RCTs, 122 people; SMD 0.54, 95% CI 0.17 to 0.91). One RCT included in the review (220 people) compared classic CBT versus interpersonal psychotherapy (see glossary, p 29) for bulimia nervosa that involved purging.[30] It found that CBT significantly improved abstinence from binge eating at the end of treatment (19 individual sessions conducted ≥ 20 wks; intention to treat analysis; 29% with CBT v 6% with interpersonal psychotherapy); however, the difference was not significant at 4, 8, and 12 months of follow up, although both groups were improved from baseline. We found two subsequent RCTs.[25,26] The first subsequent RCT (100 people with bulimia nervosa) compared dismantled CBT (with separate cognitive and behavioural components) versus full CBT versus support group only.[25] Abstinence rates were significantly higher in those receiving full CBT versus those in the support group (14/27 [52%] v 5/21 [24%]; P = 0.01; CI not provided). Abstinence rates were intermediate in those receiving a dismantled form of CBT. The second subsequent RCT (125 people with bulimia nervosa) compared four sessions of motivational enhancement therapy versus CBT.[26] It found no significant differences between the treatments. Two further analyses[28,29] found limited observational evidence that motivation and compliance factors may influence outcomes. One study[28] performed additional analyses in an RCT of CBT versus interpersonal psychotherapy.[30] It found that "stage of change", or psychological motivation and readiness to change, was not related to non-completion, but was associated with outcome in those who completed interpersonal psychotherapy. The second RCT[29] examined the effects of compliance on outcome in 62 patients randomised to guided self help or to full CBT for 16 weeks. At 6 months' follow up, but not the end of treatment, binge eating abstinence rates were greater in those who had completed two or more of the CBT exercises (chi^2 = 5.73; P = 0.04; CI not provided). **Versus antidepressants:** see option, p 26.

Harms: The RCTs did not report details of adverse effects.[22,23,26,30] The first systematic review found no significant difference in completion rates between interventions,[22] suggesting no major difference in acceptability. However, neither review could exclude infrequent serious adverse effects.[22,23] An observational study found that group psychotherapy offered very soon after presentation was sometimes perceived as threatening.[10] The subsequent RCT (100 people with bulimia nervosa) found non-completion rates were highest in those randomised to the support group as compared with those in the full CBT (11 [46%] v 3 [11%]; P = 0.006) or compared with the dismantled cognitive therapy group (11 [46%] v 4 [16%]; P = 0.019), suggesting it may be less acceptable.[22]

Comment: The first review defined CBT as psychotherapy that uses specified techniques and models,[22] but it did not define the number of sessions or specialist expertise.[31] Effect sizes for CBT were large, but over 50% of people were still binge eating at the end of treatment.[22,23] Further research is needed to evaluate the specific and non-specific effects of CBT and other psychotherapies, to explore individual characteristics (such as readiness to change) that may predict response, and to explore the long term effects of treatment. In the first review abstinence from binge eating was higher in all experimental groups, but the differences reached significance only when compared with those in a waiting list control.[22] However, waiting list or delayed treatment control groups are subject to bias because it is not possible to "blind" someone to the knowledge they are not in the active treatment group. It is difficult to interpret the clinical importance of the statistically significant changes in depression scores. It is also difficult to interpret directly the clinical importance of the benefits reported as effect sizes, where the individual RCTs used different outcomes. Further limitations are that the quality of trials was variable (e.g. 57% were not blinded).[22] Sample sizes were often small. None of the studies measured harms rigorously. The subsequent RCT of dismantled forms of CBT supports further similar studies, because it suggested that the nutritional component alone was less effective than the full CBT component alone, and this finding may have failed to reach significance because of small numbers and limited power.[25]

OPTION   OTHER PSYCHOTHERAPIES

One systematic review and one subsequent RCT have found that non-cognitive behavioural psychotherapy increases abstinence from binge eating compared with waiting list controls. The systematic review found that three specific psychotherapies other than cognitive behavioural therapy significantly reduced bulimic symptoms compared with specified control psychotherapies, but the review included RCTs with weak methods.

Benefits: **Versus waiting list controls:** We found one systematic review (search date 2002)[22] and one subsequent RCT.[32] The review also included data from studies of other binge eating (see glossary, p 29) syndromes. It found that non cognitive behavioural therapy (CBT) psychotherapies (e.g. hypnobehavioural therapy and interpersonal psychotherapy [see glossary, p 29]) versus waiting list control significantly increased abstinence from binge eating (3 RCTs, 131 people; RR 0.67, 95% CI 0.56 to 0.81) and reduced bulimia nervosa (see glossary, p 29) symptom severity measures (4 RCTs, 177 people; SMD −1.2, 95% CI −1.52 to −0.87). The additional small RCT (32 people) found that people randomised to dialectical behaviour therapy (see glossary, p 29) had significantly fewer binge eating episodes at the end of 20 sessions of treatment than did those on a waiting list (F = 30.87; P < 0.001; CI not provided).[32] **Versus a control therapy:** The systematic review reported three RCTs in which psychotherapies other than CBT were compared with a "placebo" therapy.[23] One compared nutritional counselling and stress management, one compared guided imagery and self monitoring, and the third was a three-armed RCT comparing self psychology (see glossary, p 30) (the active treatment), cognitive orientation (see glossary, p 29), and a control nutritional counselling therapy. Meta-analysis favoured the active or experimental therapies over the control therapies for reduction in bulimic symptoms (SMD = −0.51, 95% CI −1.42 to −0.51). **Versus CBT:** see option, p 23.

Harms: The RCTs did not report details of individual adverse events (see harms of CBT, p 25). Non-CBT psychotherapies include a large number of options, and it remains unclear which therapies are most effective.

Comment: The quality of trials was variable, few were blinded, sample sizes were small, and none of the studies measured harms rigorously (see comment under CBT, p 25). Waiting list or delayed treatment control groups are subject to bias because it is not possible to "blind" someone to the knowledge they are not in the active treatment group.

OPTION   ANTIDEPRESSANTS

Two systematic reviews and one subsequent RCT have found short term reduction in bulimic symptoms (significant for vomiting only in the subsequent RCT) and a small reduction in depressive symptoms. A further subsequent RCT found no signficant benefit with moclobemide 600 mg daily versus placebo, although it appeared safe.

Benefits: We found two systematic reviews,[23,33] three additional RCTs of longer term maintenance (not primary treatment studies),[34–36] and three subsequent RCTS.[27,37,38] The latter included a trial of fluoxetine in those who relapsed after psychotherapy.[37] **Versus placebo:** Both reviews found that antidepressants reduced bulimic symptoms.[23,33] The first review (search date 1998, 9 RCTs; antidepressants were imipramine [1 trial], desipramine [3 trials], phenelzine [1 trial], fluoxetine [2 trials], brofaromine [1 trial], and isocarboxazid [1 trial]) found that antidepressants versus placebo significantly reduced binge eating (see glossary, p 29) (5 RCTs; 1 imipramine, 3 desipramine, and 1 brofaromine trial; 163 people; at the end of the trials 16% were not binge eating with antidepressants; effect size weighted for sample size 0.66, 95% CI 0.52 to 0.81).[23] Antidepressants versus placebo improved purging (6 RCTs; 2 desipramine, 2 fluoxetine, 1 isocarboxazid, and 1 brofaromine trial; effect size 0.39, 95% CI 0.24 to 0.54), depression (all 9 trials; effect size 0.73, 95% CI 0.58 to 0.88), and improved scales of eating attitudes. The second review (search date 1997, 8 RCTs; antidepressants were imipramine [5 trials], amitriptyline [1 trial], desipramine [5 trials], phenelzine [2 trials], isocarboxazid [1 trial], brofaromine [1 trial], fluoxetine [5 trials], mianserin [1 trial], bupropion [1 trial], and trazodone [1 trial]) found more frequent remission of bulimic episodes with antidepressants (19% v 8% with placebo; pooled RR 0.88, 95% CI 0.83 to 0.94; NNT 9, 95% CI 6 to 16).[33] The review found no significant difference in effect between different classes of antidepressants, but there were too few trials to exclude a clinically important difference (see table 2, p 32). Fluoxetine was the only selective serotonin reuptake inhibitor included in the review, and only one trial reported remission rates.[33] Additional RCTs, two of which were not included in the above reviews, of maintenance of change in follow up[34–36] found that significantly more improvement was maintained after withdrawal of antidepressant that had been continued for 6 months.[36] However, relapse of symptoms (30–45%) over 4–6 months were high with both antidepressant and placebo.[34,35] The first subsequent RCT (22 people who relapsed following a trial of psychotherapy) compared fluoxetine versus placebo.[37] It found that more people taking fluoxetine reported 1 month of abstinence from bingeing and purging (5/13 [39%] v 0/9 [0%] taking placebo; P = 0.05; CI not provided). The second subsequent, four-armed RCT compared fluoxetine 60 mg daily versus placebo versus a self help cognitive behavioural therapy manual (see benefits of cognitive behavioural therapy, p 23) versus fluoxetine plus a self help manual (see benefits of combination treatment, p 28).[27] Those in the fluoxetine arm had significant reductions in vomiting but not in binge eating episodes. Small numbers (26 and 22 in each group, 91 subjects in total) might have limited the power of the study. Remission rates after a 16 week treatment period with fluoxetine were 16%, and were not reported for placebo. The third subsequent RCT compared moclobemide 600 mg daily versus placebo in 75 women with bulimia nervosa (see glossary, p 29).[38] Outcomes were reported for the 52 who completed the study, and active treatment was not found to be more efficacious. Remission rates were not reported. **Versus cognitive behavioural therapy:** See text, p 23. **Versus psychotherapy:** We found one systematic review (search date 1997, 5 RCTs) of antidepressants versus psychotherapy (all cognitive behavioural therapy trials), which found no significant difference in remission rates (39% with psychotherapies v 20% with antidepressants; effect size 1.28; P = 0.07; CI not provided), bulimic symptom severity (3 RCTs), or depression symptom severity at the end of the trial (3 RCTs).[39] **Versus antidepressants plus psychotherapy:** See text, p 28.

Harms: One systematic review found increased withdrawal with antidepressants than with psychotherapy (4 RCTs, 189 people; AR 40% v 18%; RR 2.18, 95% CI 1.09 to 4.35).[39] The second systematic review found significantly increased withdrawal in people taking antidepressants than with placebo (12 RCTs; 10.5% v 5.1%).[33] It found no significant difference in withdrawal due to adverse effects among and within classes of antidepressants. In pooled analysis, withdrawal due to any cause was more likely with tricyclic antidepressants than with placebo (6 RCTs; 29% v 14.4%; P = 0.01; CI not provided), but was more likely with placebo than with selective serotonin reuptake inhibitors (3 RCTs; 37% v 40%; P = 0.04; CI not provided). We found two RCTs examining specific adverse effects. One found significant increases in reclining and standing blood pulse rate, lying systolic and diastolic blood pressure, and greater orthostatic effects on blood pressure with desipramine versus placebo.[40] Cardiovascular changes were well tolerated and few people withdrew because of these effects. Meta-analysis of two double blind RCTs of fluoxetine versus placebo found no significant difference in the incidence of suicidal acts or ideation in people treated with fluoxetine versus placebo.[41] However, the overall incidence of events was low (suicide attempts 1.2%, none fatal; emergent suicidal ideation 3.1%). In addition, the fourth subsequent RCT found no differences between active and placebo groups in numbers of people withdrawing because of adverse events, and no changes in blood pressure in those on moclobemide despite reports in food diaries of a high consumption of tyramine-containing foods.[38] The third subsequent RCT failed to report on withdrawal or adverse events.[27]

Comment: We found no consistent predictors of response to treatment. Antidepressants included in the trials were imipramine, amitriptyline, desipramine, phenylzine, isocarboxazid, brofaramine, fluoxetine, mianserin, and buproprion. There is no good evidence yet for the efficacy of some "newer" antidepressants, namely venlafaxine, reboxetine, and mirtazepine. Both reviews commented on the lack of follow up.[23,33]

OPTION   COMBINATION TREATMENT

One systematic review has found that combination treatment (antidepressants plus psychotherapy) versus antidepressants alone reduces binge frequency and depressive symptoms but not remission rates. It has also found that combination treatment versus psychotherapy alone reduces short term remission and depressive symptoms but has no significant effect on binge frequency. Antidepressants alone or in combination with psychotherapy are associated with higher withdrawal rates. One subsequent study of cognitive behavioural therapy in a self help form plus fluoxetine also found reduced bulimic symptoms with combination treatment.

Benefits: We found one systematic review (search date 1997, 7 RCTs, 343 people) comparing combination treatment (antidepressants plus psychotherapy) versus either treatment alone.[42] One meta-analysis found that combined treatment with antidepressants plus psychotherapy versus antidepressants alone significantly improved binge frequency and depressive symptoms (3 RCTs, effect size 0.47; P = 0.04; CI not provided), but found no significant difference in short term remission rates (4 RCTs; 141 people; 42% with combined treatment v 23% with antidepressants alone; RR 1.38; P = 0.06; CI not provided).[42] A second meta-analysis compared psychotherapy alone versus a combination of psychotherapy plus antidepressants.[42] Combination treatment was associated with significantly higher rates of shortterm remission (6 RCTs; 257 people; 49% v 36%; RR 1.21; P = 0.03; CI not provided) and greater improvement in depressive symptoms, but no significant difference in frequency of binge eating compared with psychotherapy alone. In the subsequent RCT (see benefits of antidepressants, p 26), patients who received both the self help manual and fluoxetine 60 mg daily had the greatest reduction in bulimic symptoms, as compared with those in the placebo, fluoxetine, or self help only arms, but significance was not reported.[27] Remission rates did not differ significantly across the three active treatment arms.

Harms: Withdrawal rates were lower after psychotherapy plus antidepressants than with antidepressants alone (4 RCTs; 196 people; 34% v 41%; RR 1.19, 95% CI 0.69 to 2.05).[42] Withdrawal rates were significantly higher with psychotherapy plus antidepressants than with psychotherapy alone (6 RCTs; 295 people; 30% v 16%; RR 0.57; P = 0.01; CI not provided).[42]

Comment: None.

GLOSSARY

Binge eating Modified from DSM-IV.[1] Eating, in a discrete period (e.g. hours), a large amount of food, accompanied by a lack of control over eating during the episode.

Bulimia nervosa The American Psychiatric Association DSM-IV[1] criteria include recurrent episodes of binge eating; recurrent inappropriate compensatory behaviour to prevent weight gain; frequency of binge eating and inappropriate compensatory behaviour both, on average, at least twice a week for 3 months; self evaluation unduly influenced by body shape and weight; and disturbance occurring not exclusively during episodes of anorexia nervosa. Types of bulimia nervosa, modified from DSM-IV[1], are: purging: using self induced vomiting, laxatives, diuretics, or enemas; non-purging: fasting, exercise, but not vomiting or other abuse as for the purging type.

Cognitive behavioural therapy In bulimia nervosa this uses three overlapping phases. Phase one aims to educate the person about bulimia nervosa. People are helped to increase regularity of eating, and resist urge to binge or purge. Phase two introduces procedures to reduce dietary restraint (e.g. broadening food choices). In addition, cognitive procedures supplemented by behavioural experiments are used to identify and correct dysfunctional attitudes and beliefs, and avoidance behaviours. Phase three is the maintenance phase. Relapse prevention strategies are used to prepare for possible future set backs.[30]

Cognitive orientation therapy The cognitive orientation theory aims to generate a systematic procedure for exploring the meaning of a behaviour around themes, such as avoidance of certain emotions. Therapy for modifying behaviour focuses on systematically changing beliefs related to themes, not beliefs referring directly to eating behaviour. No attempt is made to persuade the people that their beliefs are incorrect or maladapative.[43]

Dialectical behaviour therapy A type of behavioural therapy that views emotional dysregulation as the core problem in bulimia nervosa, with binge eating and purging understood as attempts to influence, change, or control painful emotional states. Patients are taught a repertoire of skills to replace dysfunctional behaviours.[32]

Hypnobehavioural psychotherapy Uses a combination of behavioural techniques, such as self monitoring to change maladaptive eating disorders, and hypnotic techniques to reinforce and encourage behaviour change.

Interpersonal psychotherapy In bulimia nervosa this is a three phase treatment. Phase one analyses in detail the interpersonal context of the eating disorder. This leads to the formulation of an interpersonal problem area; this forms the focus of the second stage, which is aimed at helping the person make interpersonal changes. Phase three is devoted to the person's progress and an exploration of ways to handle future interpersonal difficulties. At no stage is attention paid to eating habits or body attitudes.[30]

Pure self help cognitive behavioural therapy A modified form of cognitive behavioural therapy, in which a treatment manual is provided for people to proceed with treatment on their own, or with support from a non-professional. "Guided self help" usually implies that the support person may or may not have some professional training, but is usually not a specialist in eating disorders.

Self psychology therapy This approaches bulimia nervosa as a specific case of the pathology of the self. The treated person cannot rely on people to fulfil their needs such as self esteem. They instead rely on a substance, food, to fulfill personal needs. Therapy progresses when the people move to rely on humans, starting with the therapist.[43]

REFERENCES

1. American Psychiatric Association. *Diagnostic and statistical manual of mental disorders* 4th ed. Washington DC: American Psychiatric Press, 1994.
2. Bushnell JA, Wells JE, Hornblow AR, Oakley-Brown MA, Joyce P. Prevalence of three bulimic syndromes in the general population. *Psychol Med* 1990;20:671–680.
3. Garfinkel PE, Lin B, Goering P, et al. Bulimia nervosa in a Canadian community sample: prevalence, co-morbidity, early experiences and psychosocial functioning. *Am J Psychiatry* 1995; 152:1052–1058.
4. Gard MCE, Freeman CP. The dismantling of a myth: a review of eating disorders and socioeconomic status. *Int J Eat Disord* 1996;20:1–12.
5. Hall A, Hay PJ. Eating disorder patient referrals from a population region 1977–1986. *Psychol Med* 1991;21:697–701.
6. Kendler KS, Maclean C, Neale M, et al. The genetic epidemiology of bulimia nervosa. *Am J Psychiatry* 1991;148:1627–1637.
7. Choudry IY, Mumford DB. A pilot study of eating disorders in Mirpur (Pakistan) using an Urdu version of the Eating Attitude Test. *Int J Eat Disord* 1992;11:243–251.
8. Striegel-Moore RH, Wifley DE, Caldwell MB, Needham ML, Brownell KD. Weight-related attitudes and behaviors of women who diet to lose weight: a comparison for black dieters and white dieters. *Obes Res* 1996;4:109–116.
9. Fairburn CG, Welch SL, Doll HA, Davies BA, O'Connor ME. Risk factors for bulimia nervosa: a community-based case-control study. *Arch Gen Psychiatry* 1997;54:509–517.
10. Collings S, King M. Ten year follow-up of 50 patients with bulimia nervosa. *Br J Psychiatry* 1994;164:80–87.
11. Keel PK, Mitchell JE, Miller KB, Davis TL, Crow SJ. Long-term outcome of bulimia nervosa. *Arch Gen Psychiatry* 1999;56:63–69.
12. Keel PK, Mitchell JE. Outcome in bulimia nervosa. *Am J Psychiatry* 1997;154:313–321.
13. Fairburn CG, Norman PA, Welch SL, et al. A prospective study of outcome in bulimia nervosa and the long-term effects of three psychological treatments. *Arch Gen Psychiatry* 1995;52:304–312.
14. Coker S, Vize C, Wade T, Cooper PJ. Patients with bulimia nervosa who fail to engage in cognitive behaviour therapy. *Int J Eat Disord* 1993;13:35–40.
15. Fahy TA, Russell GFM. Outcome and prognostic variables in bulimia. *Int J Eat Disord* 1993;14:135–146.
16. Rossiter EM, Agras WS, Telch CF, Schneider JA. Cluster B personality disorder characteristics predict outcome in the treatment of bulimia nervosa. *Int J Eat Disord* 1993;13:349–358.
17. Johnson C, Tobin DL, Dennis A. Differences in treatment outcome between borderline and nonborderline bulimics at 1-year follow-up. *Int J Eat Disord* 1990;9:617–627.
18. Fairburn C, Cooper Z, Doll H, Norman P, O'Conner M. The natural course of bulimia nervosa and binge eating disorder in young women. *Arch Gen Psychiatry* 2000;57:659–665.
19. Agras WS, Crow SJ, Halmi KA, Mitchell JE, Wilson GT, Kraemer HC. Outcome predictors for the cognitive behavior treatment of bulimia nervosa: data from a multisite study. *Am J Psychiatry* 2000; 157:1302–1308.
20. Reas DL, Schoemaker C, Zipfel S, Williamson DA. Prognostic value of duration of illness and early intervention in bulimia nervosa: a systematic review of the outcome literature. *Int J Eat Disord* 2001;30:1–10.
21. Lewandowski LM, Gebing TA, Anthony JL, O'Brien WH. Meta-analysis of cognitive behavioural treatment studies for bulimia. *Clin Psychol Rev* 1997;17:703–718. Search date 1995; primary sources Psychinfo and hand searches of references lists.
22. Hay PJ, Bacaltchuk J. Psychotherapy for bulimia nervosa and binging (Cochrane Review). In: The Cochrane Library, Issue 3, 2001. Oxford: Update Software. Search date 2000; primary sources Medline, Extramed, Embase, Psychlit, Current Contents, Lilacs, Scisearch, The Cochrane Controlled Trials Register 1997, The Cochrane Collaboration Depression and Anxiety Trials Register, hand search of *Int J Eat Disord* since its first issue, citation lists in identified studies and reviews, and personal contacts.
23. Whittal ML, Agras WS, Gould RA. Bulimia nervosa: a meta-analysis of psychosocial and pharmacological treatments. *Behav Ther* 1999; 30:117–135. Search date 1998; primary sources Psychlit, Medline, hand search of *Int J Eat Disord* 1990–1998, and hand search other relevant (not specified) journals and identified studies. This was reviewed in Waller G. *Evidence Based Medicine* (September/October 1999).
24. Jacobi C, Dahme B, Rustenbach S. Comparison of controlled pshco- and pharmacotherapy studies in bulimia anorexia nervosa.[in German] *Psychother Psychosom Med Psychol* 1997;47:346–364. Search date not stated; primary sources Psychological Abstracts, Medline, Psychindex, and Psychinfo.
25. Hsu LKG, Rand W, Sullivan S, et al. Cognitive therapy, nutritional therapy and their combination in the treatment of bulimia nervosa. *Psychol Med* 2001;31:871–879.
26. Treasure JL, Katzman M, Schmidt U, et al. Engagement and outcome in the treatment of bulimia nervosa: first phase of a sequential design

comparing motivation enhancement therapy and cognitive behavioural therapy. *Behav Res Ther* 1999;37:405–418.

27. Mitchell JE, Fletcher L, Hanson K, et al. The relative efficacy of fluoxetine and manual-based self-help in the treatment of outpatients with bulimia nervosa. *J Clin Psychopharmacol* 2001; 21:298–304.

28. Wolk SL, Devlin MJ. Stage of change as a predictor of response to psychotherapy for bulimia nervosa. *Int J Eat Disord* 2001;30:96–100.

29. Thiels C, Schmidt U, Troop N, Treasure J, Garthe R. Compliance with a self-care manual in guided self-change for bulimia nervosa. *Eur Eat Disord Rev* 2001;9:115–122.

30. Agras WS, Walsh BT, Fairburn CG, Wilson GT, Kraemer HC. A multicenter comparison of cognitive-behavioral therapy and interpersonal psychotherapy. *Arch Gen Psychiatry* 2000; 54:459–465.

31. Wilson GT, Fairburn CG. Treatments for eating disorders. In: Nathan PE, Gorman JM, eds. *A Guide to Treatments that Work.* New York: Oxford University Press, 1998:501–530.

32. Safer DL, Telch CF, Agras WS. Dialectical behavior therapy for bulimia nervosa. *Am J Psychiatry* 2001;158:632–634.

33. Bacaltchuk J, Hay P, Mari JJ. Antidepressants versus placebo for the treatment of bulimia nervosa: a systematic review. *Aust N Z J Psychiatry* 2000;34:310–317. Search date 1997; primary sources Medline, Extramed, Embase, Psychlit, Current Contents, Lilacs, Scisearch, The Cochrane Controlled Trials Register, The Cochrane Collaboration Depression and Anxiety Trials Register, hand search of citation lists in identified studies and reviews, and personal contact.

34. Walsh BT, Hadigan CM, Devlin MJ, Gladis M, Roose SP. Long-term outcome of antidepressant treatment for bulimia nervosa. *Am J Psychiatry* 1991;148:1206–1212.

35. Pyle RL, Mitchell JE, Eckert ED, et al. Maintenance treatment and 6-month outcome for bulimic patients who respond to initial treatment. *Am J Psychiatry* 1990;147:871–875.

36. Agras WS, Rossiter EM, Arnow B, et al. One-year follow-up of psychosocial and pharmacologic treatments for bulimia nervosa *J Clin Psychiatry* 1994;55:179–183.

37. Walsh BT, Agras WS, Devlin MJ, et al. Fluoxetine for bulimia nervosa following poor response to psychotherapy. *Am J Psychiatry* 2000;157: 1332–1334.

38. Carruba MO, Cuzzolaro M, Riva L, et al. Efficacy and tolerability of moclobemide in bulimia nervosa: a placebo-controlled trial. *Int Clin Psychopharmacol* 2001;16:27–32.

39. Bacaltchuk J, Trefiglio RP, de Oliveira IR, Lima MS, Mari JJ. Antidepressants versus psychotherapy for bulimia nervosa: a systematic review. *J Clin Pharm Ther* 1999;24:23–31. Search date 1997; primary sources Medline, Extramed, Embase, Psychlit, Current Contents, Lilacs, Scisearch, Cochrane Controlled Trials Register, Cochrane Collaboration Depression and Anxiety Trials Register, hand search of *Int J Eat Disord* since its first issue, citation lists of identified studies and reviews, and personal contacts.

40. Agras WS, Rossiter EM, Arnow B, et al. Pharmacologic and cognitive-behavioral treatment for bulimia nervosa: a controlled comparison. *Am J Psychiatry* 1992;149:82–87.

41. Wheadon DE, Rampey AH, Thompson VL, et al. Lack of association between fluoxetine and suicidality in bulimia nervosa. *J Clin Psychiatry* 1992;53:235–241.

42. Bacaltchuk J, Trefiglio RP, Oliveira IR, et al. Combination of antidepressants and psychotherapy for bulimia nervosa: a systematic review. *Acta Psychiatr Scand* 2000;101:256–264. Search date 1997; primary sources handsearch of *Int J Eat Disord* since its first issue, Medline, Extramed, Embase, Psychlit, Current Contents, Lilacs, Scisearch, Cochrane Controlled Trials Register 1997 Internet version, Cochrane Collaboration Depression and Anxiety Trials Register, hand search of all citation lists in identified studies and reviews, and personal contact.

43. Bachar E, Latzer Y, Kreitler S, Berry EM. Empirical comparison of two psychological therapies. Self psychology and cognitive orientation in the treatment of anorexia and bulimia. *J Psychother Pract Res* 1999;8:115–128.

Phillipa Hay
Psychiatrist
University of Adelaide, Adelaide, Australia

Josue Bacaltchuk
Psychiatrist
Federal University of Sao Paulo, Sao Paulo, Brazil

Competing interests: PH has received reimbursement for attending symposia from Solvay Pharmaceuticals, Bristol-Myers Squibb, and Pfizer Pharmaceuticals, and for educational training of family doctors from Bristol-Myers Squibb, Pfizer Pharmaceuticals, and Lundbeck, and has been funded by Jansenn-Cilag to attend symposia. JB has received fees from Janssen-Cilag Farmaceutica.

Bulimia nervosa

TABLE 1 Comparison of remission rates with cognitive behaviour therapy or other active psychotherapy and comparison treatment (see text, p 23).[23]

Comparison	Number of RCTs	Number of people	Absolute remission rates	RR of not remitting (95% CI)
CBT v waiting list	7	300	42% v 6%	0.64 (0.53 to 0.78)
CBT v other psychotherapy	7	474	40% v 21%	0.80 (0.61 to 1.04)
CBT v pure self help CBT	4	223	46% v 36%	0.90 (0.74 to 1.10)
Other psychotherapy v waiting list	3	131	36% v 3%	0.67 (0.56 to 0.81)

CBT, cognitive behavioural therapy.

TABLE 2 Comparison of remission rates between active drug and placebo by class of antidepressant (see text, p 27).[33]

Class: drug(s)	Number of RCTs	Number of people	RR	95% CI
TCA: desipramine, imipramine	3	132	0.86	0.7 to 1.07
SSRI: fluoxetine	1	398	0.92	0.84 to 1.01
MAOI: phenylzine, brofaramine	2	98	0.81	0.68 to 0.96
Other: bupropion, trazodone	2	87	0.86	0.76 to 0.97

MAOI, monoamine oxidase inhibitor; SSRI, selective serotonin reuptake inhibitor; TCA, tricyclic antidepressant.

INTERVENTIONS

Key Messages

- Five RCTs found insufficient evidence to support the use of antidepressants in people with chronic fatigue syndrome (CFS).
- Four RCTs found insufficient evidence to adequately assess the effects of corticosteroids in people with CFS.
- One small RCT found insufficient evidence to support the use of oral nicotinamide adenine dinucleotide in people with CFS.
- RCTs have found that a graded aerobic exercise programme or an educational intervention to encourage graded exercise improves measures of fatigue and physical functioning in people with CFS.
- We found no good evidence that prolonged rest is an effective treatment for CFS. We found indirect evidence suggesting that prolonged rest may be harmful.
- One small RCT found limited evidence of benefit from magnesium injections in people with CFS.
- One small RCT found no evidence of benefit from oral evening primrose oil in people with CFS.
- Four small RCTs of immunoglobulin G in people with CFS found only limited benefit and considerable adverse effects. RCTs of other treatments affecting the immune system found no evidence of an advantage over placebo.
- One systematic review has found that cognitive behavioural therapy administered by highly skilled therapists in specialist centres is effective in people with CFS. A subsequent multicentre RCT found that cognitive behavioural therapy may also be effective when administered by less experienced therapists.

DEFINITION Chronic fatigue syndrome (CFS) is characterised by severe, disabling fatigue and other symptoms, including musculoskeletal pain, sleep disturbance, impaired concentration, and headaches. Two widely used definitions of CFS, from the US Centers for Disease Control and Prevention[1] and from Oxford, UK,[2] were developed as operational criteria for research (see table 1, p 45). There are two important differences between these definitions. The UK criteria insist upon the presence of mental fatigue, whereas the US criteria include a requirement for several physical symptoms, reflecting the belief that CFS has an underlying immunological or infective pathology.

INCIDENCE/ PREVALENCE Community and primary care based studies have reported the prevalence of CFS to be 0–3%, depending on the criteria used.[3,4] Systematic population surveys have found similar prevalence of CFS in people of different socioeconomic status, and in all ethnic groups.[4,5]

AETIOLOGY/ RISK FACTORS The cause of CFS is poorly understood. Women are at higher risk than men (RR 1.3 to 1.7 depending on diagnostic criteria used).[6]

PROGNOSIS Studies have focused on people attending specialist clinics. A systematic review of studies of prognosis (search date 1996) found that children with CFS had better outcomes than adults: 54–94% of children showed definite improvement (after up to 6 years' follow up), whereas 20–50% of adults showed some improvement in the medium term and only 6% returned to premorbid levels of functioning.[7] Despite the considerable burden of morbidity associated with CFS, we found no evidence of increased mortality. The systematic review found that outcome was influenced by the presence of psychiatric disorders (depression and anxiety), and beliefs about causation and treatment.[7]

AIMS To reduce levels of fatigue and associated symptoms; to increase levels of activity; to improve quality of life.

OUTCOMES Severity of symptoms and their effects on physical function and quality of life. These outcomes are measured in several different ways: the medical outcomes survey short form general health survey (SF-36),[8] a rating scale measuring limitation of physical functioning caused by ill health (score range 0–100, where 0 = limited in all activities and 100 = able to carry out vigorous activities); the Karnofsky scale,[9] a modified questionnaire originally developed for the rating of quality of life in people undergoing chemotherapy for malignancy; the Beck Depression Inventory,[10] a checklist for quantifying depressive symptoms; the sickness impact profile,[11] a measure of the influence of symptoms on social and physical functioning; the Chalder fatigue scale,[12] a rating scale measuring subjective fatigue (score range 0–11, where scores ≥ 4 = excessive fatigue); the clinical global impression scale,[13] a validated measure of overall change compared with baseline at study onset, with seven possible scores from "very much worse" (score 7) to "very much better" (score 1); and self reported severity of symptoms and levels of activity, the Nottingham health profile[14] contains questions in 6 categories — energy, pain perception, sleep patterns, sense of social isolation, emotional reactions, physical mobility (weighted scores give maximum 100 for answer yes to all questions, and minimum 0 for someone with no complaints).

METHODS   *Clinical Evidence* search and appraisal November 2001.

OPTION   **ANTIDEPRESSANTS**

RCTs found insufficient evidence to support the use of antidepressants in people with chronic fatigue syndrome.

Benefits: We found one systematic review (search date 2000), which did not report quantified results.[15] **Fluoxetine:** The review identified two RCTs.[16,17] The first RCT (107 depressed and non-depressed people with chronic fatigue syndrome [CFS]) compared fluoxetine versus placebo for 8 weeks.[16] It found no significant benefit in the Beck Depression Inventory (mean difference between fluoxetine and placebo in improvement in Beck Depression Inventory −0.19, 95% CI −0.35 to −0.02), and the sickness impact profile (mean difference between fluoxetine and placebo measured by fatigue subscale of Checklist Individual Strength −0.16, 95% CI −0.64 to +0.31).[18] The second RCT (136 people with CFS) compared four groups: fluoxetine plus graded exercise; drug placebo plus graded exercise; fluoxetine plus general advice to exercise; and drug placebo plus general advice to exercise. It found no significant difference in the level of fatigue, although there were modest improvements in measures of depression at 12 weeks (Hospital Anxiety and Depression scale, mean change 1.1, 95% CI 0.03 to 2.2).[17,19] **Phenelzine:** The review identified one RCT.[15,20] The RCT (30 people with CFS) compared phenelzine versus placebo, using a modified Karnofsky scale and other outcome measures (including functional status questionnaire, profile of mood states, Centres for Epidemiological Study of Depression fatigue severity scale, and symptom severity checklist).[19] This study concluded that there was a pattern of improvement across several measures (significance tests for individual measures not carried out). **Moclobemide:** The review identified one RCT but did not report quantified results.[15,21] The RCT (90 people with CFS) compared moclobemide (450–600 mg daily) versus placebo.[21] It found that moclobemide was associated with a non-significant increase in subjectively reported global improvement (moclobemide 24/47 [51%] *v* placebo 14/43 [33%]; OR 2.16, 95% CI 0.9 to 5.1), and a non-significant improvement in the clinician rated Karnofsky scale. **Sertraline versus clomipramine:** We found one RCT comparing sertraline versus clomipramine in people with CFS.[22] It found no significant difference between sertraline and clomipramine. There was no placebo group, making it difficult to draw useful conclusions.

Harms: **Fluoxetine:** One RCT assessed separately the symptoms (which could be attributed to either CFS or to known adverse effects of fluoxetine) before starting treatment, after 2 weeks, after 6 weeks, and at the end of treatment (wk 8). It found that more people taking fluoxetine complained of tremor and perspiration compared with placebo at 8 weeks (tremor: P = 0.006; perspiration: P = 0.008).[16] It found no significant differences between fluoxetine and placebo at 2 and 6 weeks. More people taking fluoxetine withdrew from the trial because of adverse effects (9/54 [17%] v 2/53 [4%]).[16] The second RCT also found more people taking fluoxetine withdrew from the trial (24/68 people [36%] with fluoxetine withdrew v 16/69 people [24%] with placebo).[17] **Phenelzine:** Three of 15 people (20%) taking phenelzine withdrew because of adverse effects compared with none taking placebo.[20] **Sertraline versus clomipramine:** The RCT provided no information on adverse effects.[22]

Comment: Clinical trials were performed in specialist clinics. **Fluoxetine:** The first RCT[16] used a shorter duration of treatment and studied people with a longer duration of illness compared with the second RCT.[17]

OPTION   CORTICOSTEROIDS

Four RCTs provided insufficient evidence about the effects of corticosteroids in people with chronic fatigue syndrome.

Benefits: We found one systematic review (search date 2000), which did not report quantified results.[15] **Fludrocortisone:** The systematic review[15] identified two RCTs.[23,24] The first large RCT (100 people with chronic fatigue syndrome [CFS] and neurally mediated hypotension) compared fludrocortisone (titrated to 0.1 mg/daily) versus placebo for 9 weeks. It found no significant difference on a self rated global scale of "wellness" (recorded improvement of ≥ 15 points: fludrocortisone 14% v placebo 10%; P = 0.76; raw data not provided).[23] The second randomised crossover trial (20 people), which measured change in symptom severity (visual analogue scale of symptoms from 0–10 corresponding to "no problem" to "could not be worse") and functional status (using the SF-36) for 6 weeks. It found no significant difference between fludrocortisone and placebo.[24] **Hydrocortisone:** The review identified two RCTs.[15,25,26] The first RCT (65 people) compared hydrocortisone (25–35 mg/day) versus placebo for 12 weeks. It found that people taking hydrocortisone had a greater improvement in a self rated scale of "wellness" (recorded improvement of ≥ 5 points: hydrocortisone 53% v placebo 29%; P = 0.04). Other self rating scales did not show significant benefit (Beck Depression Inventory: hydrocortisone −2.1 v placebo −0.4, P = 0.17; activity scale: hydrocortisone 0.3 v placebo 0.7, P = 0.32; sickness impact profile: hydrocortisone −2.5 v placebo −2.2; P = 0.85).[25] The second randomised crossover trial (32 people) compared a lower dose of hydrocortisone (5 or 10 mg/day) versus placebo for 1 month. It found that more people taking hydrocortisone had short term improvement in fatigue (self report fatigue scale: hydrocortisone 28% v placebo 9%; results before crossover not provided).[26]

Harms: **Fludrocortisone:** In the first RCT, more people on fludrocortisone withdrew because of adverse events (12/50 [24%] v 4/50 [8%]; RR 3, 95% CI 1.04 to 8.67; NNT 6, 95% CI 3 to 8).[23] Four people withdrew from the trial because of worsening symptoms.[24]

Hydrocortisone: One RCT (using 25–35 mg/day doses of hydrocortisone) found that 12 people (40%) experienced adrenal suppression (assessed by measuring cortisol levels).[25] Another RCT (using 5 or 10 mg/day doses of hydrocortisone) reported minor adverse effects in up to 10% of participants. Three people on hydrocortisone had exacerbation of acne and nervousness, and one person on placebo had an episode of fainting.[26]

Comment: The RCTs used different reasons for their choice of active treatment. The use of fludrocortisone, a mineralocorticoid, was based on the hypothesis that CFS is associated with neurally mediated hypotension.[27] The use of hydrocortisone, a glucocorticoid, in the other RCTs was based on evidence of underactivity of the hypothalamic–pituitary–adrenocortical axis in some people with CFS.[28] Any benefit from low dose glucocorticoids seems to be short lived, and higher doses are associated with adverse effects.

OPTION   ORAL NICOTINAMIDE ADENINE DINUCLEOTIDE

One small RCT provided insufficient evidence to support the use of oral nicotinamide adenine dinucleotide in people with chronic fatigue syndrome.

Benefits: We found one systematic review (search date 2000), which did not report quantified results.[15] It identified one poor quality randomised crossover trial (35 people) comparing nicotinamide adenine dinucleotide (10 mg daily) versus placebo for 4 weeks.[29] Of the 35 people, two were excluded for non-compliance and seven were excluded for using psychotropic drugs. It found a significant improvement on a self devised 50 item symptom rating scale with nicotinamide adenine dinucleotide (8/26 people [30%] attained a 10% improvement with nicotinamide adenine dinucleotide v 2/26 people [8%] with placebo; $P < 0.05$, calculated by authors).

Harms: Minor adverse effects (loss of appetite, dyspepsia, flatulence) were reported on active treatment but did not lead to cessation of treatment.[29]

Comment: The RCT had a number of problems with its methods, including the use of inappropriate statistical analyses, the inappropriate exclusion of people from the analysis, and lack of numerical data preventing independent re-analysis of the published results.[30]

OPTION   EXERCISE

RCTs have found that a graded aerobic exercise programme or an educational intervention to encourage graded exercise improves measures of fatigue and physical functioning in people with chronic fatigue syndrome.

Benefits: We found one systematic review (search date 2000), which did not report quantified results.[15] **Aerobic exercise:** The review identified two RCTs.[15,17,31] One RCT (66 people) compared graded aerobic exercise (active intervention) versus flexibility and relaxation training (control intervention) over 12 weeks.[31] All participants undertook individual weekly sessions supervised by an exercise physiologist.

The aerobic exercise group built up their level of activity to 30 minutes of exercise a day (walking, cycling, swimming up to a maximum oxygen consumption of VO_2max 60%). People in the flexibility and relaxation training group were taught stretching and relaxation techniques (maximum 30 min/day, 5 days/wk) and were specifically told to avoid any extra physical activities. It found that more people from the aerobic exercise group reported feeling "better" or "very much better", and an improvement in physical fatigue and physical functioning versus the control group (clinical global impression scale: 52% v 27%, P = 0.04; Chalder fatigue scale: –8.4 v –3.1, P = 0.004; SF-36 scale: 20.5 v 8.0, P = 0.01). The flexibility training group crossed over to aerobic exercise at the end of the trial and significant improvements from baseline were found (peak oxygen consumption; P < 0.0001: physical function; P = 0.002 compared with baseline). The second RCT (136 people) compared four groups (graded aerobic exercise plus fluoxetine; graded aerobic exercise plus drug placebo; general advice plus fluoxetine; general advice plus drug placebo) over 24 weeks.[17] The graded exercise groups were given specific advice to undertake preferred aerobic exercise (such as walking, jogging, swimming, or cycling) for 20 minutes three times a week up to an energy expenditure of 75% of VO_2max. The general advice (exercise placebo) groups were not given any specific advice on frequency, intensity, or duration of aerobic activity they should be undertaking. It found that, at week 26, there were fewer cases of fatigue in the graded exercise groups versus people receiving general advice (Chalder fatigue scale < 4: 12/67 [18%] v 4/69 [6%]; RR 3.1, 95% CI 1.05 to 9.10; NNT 9, 95% CI 5 to 91). **Educational intervention:** The review identified one RCT (148 people) but did not report quantified results.[15,32] The RCT compared three types of educational interventions to encourage graded exercise versus only providing written information (control group).[32] The participants in the three educational intervention groups received two treatment sessions, two telephone follow ups, and an educational package that provided an explanation of symptoms and encouraged home based exercise. One group received seven additional follow up telephone calls and another received seven additional face to face sessions over 4 months. People in the written information group received advice and an information booklet that encouraged graded activity but gave no explanation for the symptoms. It found that, in people who had received an educational intervention, there was improvement in physical functioning, fatigue, mood, sleep, and disability (self reported) compared with the people who had only received written information. No significant differences were found between the educational intervention groups (mean for 3 educational intervention groups versus written information, SF-36 subscale: ≥ 25 or an increase of ≥ 10, 1 year after randomisation, 69% v 6%, P < 0.001; Chalder fatigue scale: 3 v 10, P < 0.001; Hospital Anxiety and Depression scale: depression 4 v 10, P < 0.001; anxiety 7 v 10, P < 0.01).

Harms: None of the RCTs reported data on adverse effects, and we found no evidence that exercise is harmful in people with chronic fatigue syndrome. In the second aerobic exercise RCT, more people withdrew with exercise than without exercise but the difference was not quite significant (25/68 [37%] with exercise v 15/69 [22%] without exercise; RR 1.7, 95% CI 0.98 to 2.9).[17] The reasons for the withdrawals from the graded exercise groups were not stated.

Comment: Experience suggests that symptoms of chronic fatigue syndrome may be exacerbated by overly ambitious or overly hasty attempts at exercise.

OPTION   PROLONGED REST

We found no good evidence that prolonged rest is an effective treatment for chronic fatigue syndrome. We found indirect evidence suggesting that prolonged rest may be harmful.

Benefits: We found no systematic review or RCTs of prolonged rest in people with chronic fatigue syndrome.

Harms: We found no direct evidence of harmful effects of rest in people with chronic fatigue syndrome. We found observational evidence suggesting that prolonged inactivity may perpetuate or worsen fatigue and is associated with symptoms in both healthy volunteers[33] and in people recovering from viral illness.[34]

Comment: It is not clear that evidence from people recovering from viral illness can be extrapolated to people with chronic fatigue syndrome.

OPTION   MAGNESIUM SUPPLEMENTS

One small RCT found limited evidence of benefit from magnesium injections.

Benefits: We found one systematic review (search date 2000), which did not report quantified results.[15] The review identified one RCT (32 people with chronic fatigue syndrome), which compared weekly intramuscular injections of magnesium sulphate 50% versus placebo (water for injection) for 6 weeks.[35] It found benefits with magnesium in terms of measures of overall benefit (12/15 [80%] v 3/17 [18%]; RR 4.5, 95% CI 1.6 to 13.1; NNT 2, 95% CI 2 to 4), energy (P = 0.002), pain (P = 0.001), and emotional reactions (P = 0.013).

Harms: The RCT reported no adverse effects.

Comment: Subsequent studies have not found a deficiency of magnesium in people with chronic fatigue syndrome.[36–38] In the RCT, only red blood cell magnesium was slightly lower than the normal range. In the three subsequent studies, magnesium was in the normal range and no different from controls. However, none of the studies state where the normal range comes from so it is difficult to say if they are equivalent.

OPTION   EVENING PRIMROSE OIL

One small RCT of evening primrose oil found no evidence of benefit.

Benefits: We found one systematic review (search date 2000), which did not report quantified results.[15] The review identified one RCT (50 people with chronic fatigue syndrome according to Oxford, UK, diagnostic criteria), which compared evening primrose oil (4 g/day) versus placebo for 3 months.[39] It found no significant difference between groups in depression scores (Beck Depression Inventory), physical symptoms, or patient assessment (at 3 months 46% were improved with placebo v 29% with evening primrose oil; P = 0.09; figures were not presented in a manner that allowed RR with CI to be calculated).

Harms: The RCT reported no adverse effects.

Comment: One RCT (63 people) compared evening primrose oil (4 g/day) versus placebo in people with a diagnosis of postviral fatigue syndrome.[40] This diagnosis was made on the basis of overwhelming fatigue, myalgia, and depression, which had been present for at least 1 year and all had been preceded by a febrile illness. At 3 months, 33/39 (85%) of the people on active treatment had improved compared with 4/24 (17%) on placebo — a significant benefit (P < 0.0001). The difference in outcome may be partly explained by participant selection; the study in people with chronic fatigue syndrome used currently accepted diagnostic criteria.[39] Also, whereas this RCT used liquid paraffin as a placebo,[40] the chronic fatigue syndrome RCT used sunflower oil, which is better tolerated and less likely to affect the placebo response adversely.[39]

| OPTION | IMMUNOTHERAPY |

Four small RCTs of immunoglobulin G in people with chronic fatigue syndrome found limited benefit and considerable adverse effects. RCTs of other treatments affecting the immune system found no evidence of a benefit over placebo.

Benefits: We found one systematic review (search date 2000), which did not report quantified results.[15] **Immunoglobulin G:** The review identified four relevant RCTs comparing immunoglobulin G versus placebo for 6 months.[41–44] The first RCT (30 people) compared monthly intravenous injections of immunoglobulin G (1 g/kg) versus placebo (albumin).[41] After 6 months, no large differences were found in measures of fatigue (self reported symptom severity) or in physical and social functioning (SF-36). There was a significant improvement in social function with placebo versus immunoglobulin G (dichotomous figures not provided). The second RCT (49 people) compared monthly intravenous immunoglobulin G (2 g/kg) versus intravenous placebo (a maltose solution) for 3 months.[42] More people receiving immunoglobulin G versus placebo improved in terms of a physician rated assessment of symptoms and disability (10/23 [44%] v 3/26 [11%]; P = 0.03). The second RCT (99 adults) compared placebo versus three doses of immunoglobulin G (0.5, 1, or 2 g/kg).[43] It found no significant difference in quality of life, scores on visual analogue scales, or in changes in hours spent in non-sedentary activities. The third RCT (71 adolescents aged 11–18 years) compared immunoglobulin G (1 g/kg) versus placebo.[44] Three infusions were given 1 month apart. There was a significant difference between the active treatment and control groups in mean functional outcome, which was determined by taking the mean of clinician ratings from four areas of the participants' activities (number of people achieving improvement of

≥ 25% at 6 months: 26/36 [52%] with immunoglobin v 15/34 [31%] with placebo, RR 1.6, 95% CI 1.1 to 2.5). However, both groups showed significant improvements from baseline, continuing to the 6 month assessment after treatment. **Other treatments:** The review identified two RCTs (30 people) comparing interferon alfa versus placebo.[45,46] The first RCT only found treatment benefit on subgroup analysis of people with isolated natural killer cell dysfunction.[45] The second randomised crossover trial did not present results in a manner that allowed clear interpretation of treatment effect.[46] Other RCTs found no significant advantage over placebo from aciclovir,[47] dialysable leucocyte extract (in a factorial design with cognitive behavioural therapy),[48] or terfenadine.[49]

Harms:
Immunoglobulin G: In the first RCT, adverse effects judged to be worse than pretreatment symptoms in either group included gastro-intestinal complaints (18 people), headaches (23 people), arthralgia (6 people), and worsening fatigue. Of these symptoms, only headaches differed significantly between the groups (immunoglobulin G 14/15 [93%] v placebo 9/15 [60%]). Six participants (3 immunoglobulin G, 3 placebo) were considered to have major adverse effects. Adverse events by treatment group were only reported for headache.[41] **Other treatments:** In the RCT comparing interferon alfa 2/13 (15%) people taking active treatment developed neutropenia.[45]

Comment:
Immunoglobulin G: The first two RCTs differed in that the second used twice the dose of immunoglobulin G, did not require that participants fulfil the operational criteria (similar but not identical to US Centers for Disease Control and Prevention criteria) for chronic fatigue syndrome, and made no assessments of them during the study, waiting until 3 months after completion.[42] **Other treatments:** Terfenadine, particularly at high blood concentrations, is associated with rare hazardous cardiac arrhythmias.[50]

OPTION	COGNITIVE BEHAVIOURAL THERAPY

One systematic review has found that cognitive behavioural therapy administered by highly skilled therapists in specialist centres is effective in people with chronic fatigue syndrome. One additional multicentre RCT has found that cognitive behavioural therapy may also be effective when administered by less experienced therapists.

Benefits:
We found two systematic reviews (search dates 2000 and 1998).[15,51] The first review[51] identified three RCTs that met the reviewers' inclusion criteria (all participants fulfilled accepted diagnostic criteria for chronic fatigue syndrome [CFS], use of adequate randomisation, and use of controls).[48,52,53] The second review identified one additional RCT that met our inclusion criteria but the review did not report quantified results.[16,54] The first RCT (90 people with CFS according to Australian diagnostic criteria that are similar to US Centers for Disease Control and Prevention [CDC] criteria) evaluated cognitive behavioural therapy (CBT) and immunological therapy (dialysable leucocyte extract) using a factorial design.[48] The comparison group received standard medical care. It found no significant difference in quality of life measures

Chronic fatigue syndrome

(Karnofsky scale and symptom report on a visual analogue scale) between CBT and standard medical care. CBT was given every 2 weeks for six sessions lasting 30–60 minutes each. Treatment involved encouraging participants to exercise at home and feel less helpless. The second RCT (60 people with CFS according to Oxford, UK, diagnostic criteria) compared CBT versus normal general practice care in people attending a secondary care centre.[53] It found that, at 12 months, CBT improved quality of life (Karnofsky scale) compared with those receiving standard medical care (final score >80 22/30 [73%] with CBT v 8/30 [27%] with placebo; RR 2.75, 95% CI 1.54 to 5.32; NNT 3, 95% CI 2 to 5). The active treatment consisted of a cognitive behavioural assessment, followed by 16 weekly sessions of behavioural experiments, problem solving activity, and re-evaluation of thoughts and beliefs inhibiting return to normal functioning. The third RCT (60 people with CFS according to CDC diagnostic criteria in people attending a secondary care centre) compared CBT with relaxation treatment.[52] It found substantial improvement in physical functioning (based on predefined absolute or relative increases in the SF-36 score) with CBT compared with relaxation treatment (19/30 [63%] with CBT v 5/30 [17%] with relaxation; RR 3.7, 95% CI 2.37 to 6.31; NNT 3, 95% CI 1 to 7). Improvement continued over 6–12 months' follow up. CBT was given in 13 weekly sessions. A 5 year follow up study of 53 (88%) of the original participants found that more people rated themselves as "much improved" or "very much improved" with CBT compared with relaxation treatment (17/25 [68%] with CBT v 10/28 [36%] with relaxation treatment; RR 1.9, 95% CI 1.1 to 3.4; NNT 4, 95% CI 2 to 19).[55] More people treated with CBT met the authors' criteria for complete recovery at 5 years but the difference was not significant (17/31 [55%] with CBT v 7/22 [32%] with relaxation treatment; RR 1.7, 95% CI 0.9 to 3.4). The subsequent multicentre RCT (278 people with CFS according to CDC criteria) compared CBT, guided support groups, or no intervention.[54] The CBT consisted of 16 sessions over 8 months administered by 13 therapists with no previous experience of treating CFS. The guided support groups were similar to CBT in terms of treatment schedule, with the participants receiving non-directive support from a social worker. At 8 months' follow up it found that more people in the CBT group met the criteria for clinical improvement for fatigue severity (checklist individual strength) and self reported improvement in fatigue compared with the guided support and no treatment groups (fatigue severity: CBT v support group, 27/83 [33%] v 10/80 [13%], RR 2.6, 95% CI 1.3 to 5.0; CBT v no intervention 27/83 [33%] v 8/62 [13%], RR 2.5, 95% CI 1.2 to 5.2; self reported improvement: CBT v support group 42/74 [57%] v 12/71 [17%], RR 3.4, 95% CI 1.9 to 5.8; CBT v no intervention 42/74 [57%] v 23/78 [30%], RR 1.9, 95% CI 1.3 to 2.9). The results were not corrected for multiple comparisons.

Harms: No harmful effects were reported.

Comment: The effectiveness of CBT for CFS outside of specialist settings has been questioned. The results of the multicentre RCT suggest that cognitive behavioural therapy may be effective when administered by less experienced therapists given adequate supervision. The trial had a high withdrawal rate (25% after 8 months), especially in the CBT and guided support groups. Although the presented confidence intervals are not adjusted for multiple comparisons the results would remain significant after any reasonable adjustment. The authors comment that the results were similar following intention to treat analysis but these results were not presented.[54] A randomised trial comparing CBT and non-directive counselling found that both interventions were of benefit in the management of people consulting their family doctor because of fatigue symptoms. In this study, 28% of the sample conformed to CDC criteria for CFS.[56]

REFERENCES

1. Fukuda K, Straus S, Hickie I, et al. The chronic fatigue syndrome: a comprehensive approach to its definition and study. *Ann Intern Med* 1994; 121:953–959.

2. Sharpe M, Archard LC, Banatvala JE. A report — chronic fatigue syndrome: guidelines for research. *J R Soc Med* 1991;84:118–121.

3. Wessely S, Chalder T, Hirsch S, et al. The prevalence and morbidity of chronic fatigue and chronic fatigue syndrome: a prospective primary care study. *Am J Public Health* 1997;87: 1449–1455.

4. Steele L, Dobbins JG, Fukuda K, et al. The epidemiology of chronic fatigue in San Francisco. *Am J Med* 1998;105(suppl 3A):83–90.

5. Lawrie SM, Pelosi AJ. Chronic fatigue syndrome in the community: prevalence and associations. *Br J Psychiatry* 1995;166:793–797.

6. Wessely S. The epidemiology of chronic fatigue syndrome. *Epidemiol Rev* 1995;17:139–151.

7. Joyce J, Hotopf M, Wessely S. The prognosis of chronic fatigue and chronic fatigue syndrome: a systematic review. *QJM* 1997;90:223–133. Search date 1996; primary sources Medline, Embase, Current Contents, and Psychlit.

8. Stewart AD, Hays RD, Ware JE. The MOS short-form general health survey. *Med Care* 1988;26: 724–732.

9. Karnofsky DA, Burchenal JH, MacLeod CM. *The clinical evaluation of chemotherapeutic agents in cancer.* New York Academy of Medicine, New York: Columbia University Press; 1949:191–206.

10. Beck AT, Ward CH, Mendelson M, Mock JE, Erbaugh JK. An inventory for measuring depression. *Arch Gen Psychiatry* 1961;4:561–571.

11. Bergner M, Bobbit RA, Carter WB, et al. The sickness impact profile: development and final revision of a health status measure. *Med Care* 1981;19:787–805.

12. Chalder T, Berelowitz C, Pawlikowska T. Development of a fatigue scale. *J Psychosom Res* 1993;37:147–154.

13. Guy W. *ECDEU assessment manual for psychopharmacology.* Rockville, MD: National Institute of Mental Health, 1976:218–222.

14. Hunt SM, McEwen J, McKenna SP. Measuring health status: a new tool for clinicians and epidemiologists. *J Roy Coll Gen Prac* 1985,35: 185–188.

15. Whiting P, Bagnall A-M, Sowden A, et al. Interventions for the treatment and management of chronic fatigue syndrome: A systematic review. *JAMA* 2001;286:1360–1368. Search date 2000; primary sources Medline, Embase, Psychlit, ERIC, Current Contents, Internet searches, bibliographies from the retrieved references, individuals and organisations through a web site dedicated to the review, and members of advisory panels.

16. Vercoulen J, Swanink C, Zitman F. Randomised, double-blind, placebo-controlled study of fluoxetine in chronic fatigue syndrome. *Lancet* 1996;347:858–861.

17. Wearden AJ, Morriss RK, Mullis R, et al. Randomised, double-blind, placebo controlled treatment trial of fluoxetine and a graded exercise programme for chronic fatigue syndrome. *Br J Psychiatry* 1998;172:485–490.

18. Vercoulen JHMM, Swanink CMA, Galama JMD, Fennis JFM, van der Meer JWM, Bleijenberg G. Dimensional assessment of chronic fatigue syndrome. *J Psychosom Res* 1994;38:383–392.

19. Zigmond AS, Snaith RP. The Hospital Anxiety and Depression Scale (HAD). *Acta Psychiatr Scand* 1983;67:361–370.

20. Natelson BH, Cheu J, Pareja J, et al. Randomised, double blind, controlled placebo-phase in trial of low dose phenelzine in the chronic fatigue syndrome. *Psychopharmacology* 1996;124: 226–230.

21. Hickie IB, Wilson AJ, Murray Wright J, Bennett BK, Wakefield D, Lloyd AR. A randomized, double-blind, placebo-controlled trial of moclobemide in patients with chronic fatigue syndrome. *J Clin Psychiatry* 2000;61:643–648.

22. Behan PO, Hannifah H. 5-HT reuptake inhibitors in CFS. *J Immunol Immunopharmacol* 1995;15: 66–69.

23. Rowe PC, Calkins H, DeBusk K, et al. Fludrocortisone acetate to treat neurally mediated hypotension in chronic fatigue syndrome. *JAMA* 2001;285:52–59.

24. Peterson PK, Pheley A, Schroeppel J, et al. A preliminary placebo-controlled crossover trial of fludrocortisone for chronic fatigue syndrome. *Arch Intern Med* 1998;158:908–914.

25. McKenzie R, O'Fallon A, Dale J, et al. Low-dose hydrocortisone for treatment of chronic fatigue syndrome. *JAMA* 1998;280:1061–1066.

26. Cleare AJ, Heap E, Malhi G, et al. Low-dose hydrocortisone in chronic fatigue syndrome: a randomised crossover trial. *Lancet* 1999;353: 455–458.

27. Bou-Holaigah I, Rowe P, Kan J, et al. The relationship between neurally mediated hypotension and the chronic fatigue syndrome. *JAMA* 1995;274:961–967.

28. Demitrack M, Dale J, Straus S, et al. Evidence for impaired activation of the hypothalamic-pituitary-adrenal axis in patients with chronic fatigue syndrome. *J Clin Endocrinol Metab* 1991;73: 1224–1234.

29. Forsyth LM, Preuss HG, MacDowell AL, et al. Therapeutic effects of oral NADH on the symptoms of patients with chronic fatigue syndrome. *Ann Allergy Asthma Immunol* 1999;82:185–191.

30. Colquhoun D, Senn S. Re: Therapeutic effects of oral NADH on the symptoms of patients with chronic fatigue syndrome. *Ann Allergy Asthma Immunol* 2000;84:639–640.

31. Fulcher KY, White PD. A randomised controlled trial of graded exercise therapy in patients with the chronic fatigue syndrome. *BMJ* 1997;314: 1647–1652.

32. Powell P, Bentall RP, Nye FJ, Edwards RHT. Randomised controlled trial of patient education to encourage graded exercise in chronic fatigue syndrome. *BMJ* 2001;322:387–390.

33. Sandler H, Vernikos J. *Inactivity: physiological effects*. London: Academic Press, 1986.

34. Dalrymple W. Infectious mononucleosis: 2. Relation of bed rest and activity to prognosis. *Postgrad Med* 1961;35:345–349.

35. Cox IM, Campbell MJ, Dowson D. Red blood cell magnesium and chronic fatigue syndrome. *Lancet* 1991;337:757–760.

36. Clague JE, Edwards RHT, Jackson MJ. Intravenous magnesium loading in chronic fatigue syndrome. *Lancet* 1992;340:124–125.

37. Hinds G, Bell NP, McMaster D, et al. Normal red cell magnesium concentrations and magnesium loading tests in patients with chronic fatigue syndrome. *Ann Clin Biochem* 1994;31:459–461.

38. Swanink CM, Vercoulen JH, Bleijenberg G, et al. Chronic fatigue syndrome: a clinical and laboratory study with a well matched control group. *J Intern Med* 1995;237:499–506.

39. Warren G, McKendrick M, Peet M. The role of essential fatty acids in chronic fatigue syndrome. *Acta Neurol Scand* 1999;99:112–116.

40. Behan PO, Behan WMH, Horrobin D. Effect of high doses of essential fatty acids on the postviral fatigue syndrome. *Acta Neurol Scand* 1990;82: 209–216.

41. Peterson PK, Shepard J, Macres M, et al. A controlled trial of intravenous immunoglobulin G in chronic fatigue syndrome. *Am J Med* 1990;89: 554–560.

42. Lloyd A, Hickie I, Wakefield D, et al. A double-blind, placebo-controlled trial of intravenous immunoglobulin therapy in patients with chronic fatigue syndrome. *Am J Med* 1990;89:561–568.

43. Vollmer-Conna U, Hickie I, Hadzi-Pavlovic D, et al. Intravenous immunoglobulin is ineffective in the treatment of patients with chronic fatigue syndrome. *Am J Med* 1997;103:38–43.

44. Rowe KS. Double-blind randomized controlled trial to assess the efficacy of intravenous gammaglobulin for the management of chronic fatigue syndrome in adolescents. *J Psychiatr Res* 1997;31:133–147.

45. See DM, Tilles JG. Alpha interferon treatment of patients with chronic fatigue syndrome. *Immunol Invest* 1996;25:153–164.

46. Brook M, Bannister B, Weir W. Interferon-alpha therapy for patients with chronic fatigue syndrome. *J Infect Dis* 1993;168:791–792.

47. Straus SE, Dale JK, Tobi M, et al. Acyclovir treatment of the chronic fatigue syndrome. Lack of efficacy in a placebo-controlled trial. *N Engl J Med* 1988;319:1692–1698.

48. Lloyd A, Hickie I, Boughton R, et al. Immunologic and psychological therapy for patients with chronic fatigue syndrome. *Am J Med* 1993;94:197–203.

49. Steinberg P, McNutt BE, Marshall P, et al. Double-blind placebo-controlled study of efficacy of oral terfenadine in the treatment of chronic fatigue syndrome. *J Allergy Clin Immunol* 1996;97: 119–126.

50. Medicines Control Agency (UK). *Current Problems in Pharmacovigilance*, Volume 23, September 1997.

51. Price JR, Couper J. Cognitive behaviour therapy for CFS. In: The Cochrane Library, Issue 4, 2001. Oxford: Update Software. Search date 1998; primary sources Medline, Embase, Biological Abstracts, Sigle, Index to Theses of Great Britain and Ireland, Index to Scientific and Technical Proceedings, Science Citation Index, Trials Register of the Depression, Anxiety and Neurosis Group, citation lists, and personal contacts.

52. Deale A, Chalder T, Marks I, et al. Cognitive behaviour therapy for chronic fatigue syndrome: a randomized controlled trial. *Am J Psychiatry* 1997; 154:408–414.

53. Sharpe M, Hawton K, Simkin S, et al. Cognitive behaviour therapy for chronic fatigue syndrome: a randomized controlled trial. *BMJ* 1996;312: 22–26.

54. Prins JB, Bleijenberg G, Bazelmans E, et al. Cognitive behaviour therapy for chronic fatigue syndrome: a multicentre randomised controlled trial. *Lancet* 2001;357:841–847.

55. Deale A, Husain K, Chalder T, Wessely S. Long-term outcome of cognitive behaviour therapy versus relaxation therapy for chronic fatigue syndrome: a 5-year follow-up study. *Am J Psychiatry* 2001;158:2038–2042.

56. Ridsdale L, Godfrey E, Chalder T, et al. Chronic fatigue in general practice: is counselling as good as cognitive behaviour therapy? A UK randomised trial. *Br J Gen Pract* 2001;51:19–24.

Steven Reid
Clinical Research Fellow

Trudie Chalder
Reader

Anthony Cleare
Senior Lecturer

Matthew Hotopf
Senior Lecturer

Simon Wessely
Professor of Epidemiological and Liaison Psychiatry

Guy's, King's and St Thomas' School of Medicine and Institute of Psychiatry
London
UK

Competing interests: None declared.

TABLE 1	Diagnostic criteria for chronic fatigue syndrome (see text, p 34).

CDC 1994[1]

Clinically evaluated, medically unexplained fatigue of at least 6 months' duration that is:

- of new onset
- not a result of ongoing exertion
- not substantially alleviated by rest
- a substantial reduction in previous levels of activity

The occurrence of four or more of the following symptoms:

- subjective memory impairment
- tender lymph nodes
- muscle pain
- joint pain
- headache
- unrefreshing sleep
- postexertional malaise (> 24 h)

Oxford, UK[2]

Severe, disabling fatigue of at least 6 months' duration that:

- affects both physical and mental functioning
- was present for more than 50% of the time

Other symptoms, particularly myalgia, sleep, and mood disturbance, may be present.

Exclusion criteria

- Active, unresolved, or suspected disease likely to cause fatigue
- Psychotic, melancholic, or bipolar depression (but not uncomplicated major depression)
- Psychotic disorders
- Dementia
- Anorexia or bulimia nervosa
- Alcohol or other substance misuse
- Severe obesity

- Active, unresolved, or suspect disease likely to cause fatigue
- Psychotic, melacholic, or bipolar depression (but not uncomplicated major depression)
- Psychotic disorders
- Dementia
- Anorexia or bulimia nervosa

CDC, US Centers for Disease Control and Prevention

Dementia

Search date June 2001

James Warner and Rob Butler

INTERVENTIONS

Key Messages

- Most RCTs use proxy outcomes, such as cognitive function, rather than outcomes likely to be important to people with dementia and their carers, such as activities of daily living and quality of life. People in dementia studies are often not representative of people in routine settings. Few studies are in primary care.

- Systematic reviews and RCTs have found:
  - Improved cognitive function and global clinical state with donepezil 10 mg daily versus placebo, with few adverse effects.
  - Improved cognitive function but frequent nausea with rivastigmine 6–12 mg.
  - Improved cognitive function with galantamine at both 24 and 32 mg, but 24 mg dose is better tolerated.
  - Limited evidence that tacrine improves cognitive function or behaviour, but is associated with hepatotoxicity.
  - Improved cognition with slow release physostigmine, but adverse effects were common.
  - Insufficient evidence about nicotine.
  - No evidence of benefit with lecithin.
  - Conflicting evidence about the effects of non-steroidal anti-inflammatory drugs.
  - Some evidence of benefit from oestrogen (in women).
  - Improved cognitive function and few adverse effects with Ginkgo biloba 120 mg daily.
  - No evidence of benefit from vitamin E.
  - Selegiline versus placebo improves cognitive function, behaviour, and mood, with few adverse effects. No evidence was found of an effect on clinical global state.
  - Insufficient evidence about reminiscence therapy.
  - Reality orientation versus no treatment improves cognitive function and behaviour.
  - Weak evidence that music therapy may be beneficial in people with dementia.
  - Risperidone and olanzapine produce a small but significant improvement of behavioural disorders.
  - No significant improvement with haloperidol compared with placebo.
  - Carbamazepine and sodium valproate improved behavioural symptoms compared with placebo.
  - No evidence of benefit with trazodone compared with placebo or haloperidol.
  - Conflicting evidence about behaviour management.

DEFINITION   **Dementia** is characterised by chronic, global, non-reversible impairment of cerebral function. It usually results in loss of memory (initially of recent events), loss of executive function (such as the ability to make decisions or sequence complex tasks), and changes in personality. **Alzheimer's disease** is a type of dementia characterised by an insidious onset and slow deterioration, and involves speech, motor, personality, and executive function impairment. It should be diagnosed after other systemic, psychiatric, and neurological causes of dementia have been excluded clinically and by laboratory investigation. **Vascular dementia** (multi-infarct dementia) is a stepwise deterioration of executive function with or without language and motor dysfunction occurring as a result of cerebral arterial occlusion. It usually occurs in the presence of vascular risk factors (diabetes, hypertension, and smoking). Characteristically, it has a more sudden onset and stepwise progression than Alzheimer's disease. **Lewy body dementia** is an insidious impairment of executive functions with (1) Parkinsonism, (2) visual hallucinations, and (3) fluctuating cognitive abilities and increased risk of falls or autonomic failure.[1,2] Careful clinical examination of people with mild to moderate dementia, and the use of established diagnostic criteria, has an antemortem positive predictive value of 70–90% compared with the gold standard of postmortem diagnosis.[3,4]

INCIDENCE/ PREVALENCE About 6% of people aged over 65 years and 30% of people aged over 90 years have some form of dementia.[5] Dementia is rare before the age of 60 years. The most common types of dementia are Alzheimer's disease, vascular dementia, mixed vascular and Alzheimer's disease, and Lewy body dementia. Alzheimer's disease and vascular dementia (including mixed dementia) are each estimated to account for 35–50% of dementia, and Lewy body dementia is estimated to account for up to 20% of dementia in the elderly, varying with geographical, cultural, and racial factors.[1,5-10]

AETIOLOGY/ RISK FACTORS The cause of Alzheimer's disease is unclear. A key pathological process is deposition of abnormal amyloid in the central nervous system.[11] Most people with the relatively rare condition of early onset Alzheimer's disease (before age 60 years) show an autosomal dominant inheritance due to mutations on presenelin or amyloid precursor protein genes. Several genes (*APP*, *PS-1*, and *PS-2*) have been identified. Later onset dementia is sometimes clustered in families, but specific gene mutations have not been identified. Head injury, Down's syndrome, and lower premorbid intellect may be risk factors for Alzheimer's disease. Vascular dementia is related to cardiovascular risk factors, such as smoking, hypertension, and diabetes. The aetiology of Lewy body dementia is unknown. Brain acetylcholine activity is reduced in many forms of dementia, and the level of reduction correlates with cognitive impairment. Many treatments for Alzheimer's disease enhance cholinergic activity.[1,6]

PROGNOSIS Alzheimer's disease usually has an insidious onset with progressive reduction in cerebral function. Diagnosis is difficult in the early stages. Average life expectancy after diagnosis is 7–10 years.[10] People with Lewy body dementia have an average life expectancy of around 6 years after diagnosis.[5] Behavioural problems, depression, and psychotic symptoms are common in all types of dementia.[12,13] Eventually, most people with dementia find it difficult to perform simple tasks without help.

AIMS To improve cognitive function (memory, orientation, attention, and concentration); to reduce behavioural and psychological symptoms (wandering, aggression, anxiety, depression, and psychosis); to improve quality of life for both the individual and carer, with minimum adverse effects.

OUTCOMES Quality of life of the person with dementia and their carer (rarely used in clinical trials). Comprehensive scales of cognitive function (e.g. Alzheimer's Disease Assessment Scale cognitive subscale [ADAS-cog], 70 point scale, lower scores signify better function;[14] Mini Mental State Examination [MMSE], 30 point scale, higher scores signify better function[15]). ADAS-cog is more sensitive than MMSE, but neither scale directly reflects outcomes important to people with dementia or their carers. A 7 point change in the ADAS-cog has been regarded as clinically important. Measures of global state (e.g. clinician interview based impression of change with caregiver input scale, Clinician's Interview Based Impression of

Change-Plus: 7 points). Measures of psychiatric symptoms (e.g. Neuropsychiatric Inventory, maximum score 144, higher scores indicate greater difficulties; Dementia Mood Assessment Scale; and Brief Psychiatric Rating Scale, which use lower scores to signify improved symptoms; Behave-AD scale, scores 0–75, lower scores indicate better function); time to institutionalisation or death (rarely reported because of the short duration of most trials).[16]

METHODS *Clinical Evidence* search and appraisal June 2001.

QUESTION	What are the effects of treatments on cognition?

OPTION	DONEPEZIL

One systematic review has found that donepezil versus placebo improves cognitive function and is well tolerated. We found no evidence that donepezil significantly improved quality of life. We found no RCTs of donepezil in vascular dementia or Lewy body dementia.

Benefits: **Alzheimer's disease:** We found one systematic review of donepezil (search date 2000, 8 RCTs of 12, 24, and 52 wks duration, 2664 people with mild or moderate Alzheimer's disease).[17] Five RCTs reported results using the Alzheimer's Disease Assessment Scale cognitive subscale (ADAS-cog); three of 12 weeks' duration and two of 24 weeks' duration. The review found that donepezil 10 mg daily versus placebo significantly improved cognitive function in RCTs of 24 weeks[1] duration (821 people; ADAS-cog: WMD −2.9, 95% CI −3.7 to −2.2; Mini Mental State Examination [MMSE]: WMD 1.4, 95% CI 0.7 to 2.1) (see table 1, p 65), and global clinical state (Clinician's Interview Based Session Impression of Change: OR 0.5, 95% CI 0.3 to 0.7), but did not significantly improve patient or carer rated quality of life. One large RCT in the review (24 wks, double blind, 473 people with mild to moderate Alzheimer's disease) of donepezil 10 mg daily versus placebo found that the number of people needing treatment for one person to have clinically important improvement in cognitive function was 6 (NNT 4 for a 4 point improvement in ADAS-cog; NNT 6 for a 7 point improvement).[20] Another RCT over 52 weeks (286 people) found donepezil 10 mg daily versus placebo significantly improved cognitive function (MMSE: WMD 1.7, 95% CI 0.8 to 2.6) and activities of daily living. An unblinded extension of an RCT observed 133 people on donepezil 3–10 mg daily for up to 240 weeks.[21] Improved cognitive function compared with baseline was present for 38 weeks, and cognitive function remained above the level throughout the period of observation. **Vascular dementia:** We found no systematic review or RCTs relating to donepezil treatment and it's effect on cognitive function in vascular dementia. **Lewy body dementia:** We found no systematic review and no RCTs relating to donepezil treatment and it's effect on cognitive function in Lewy body dementia.

Harms: Adverse effects common to all cholinesterase inhibitors include anorexia, nausea, vomiting, and diarrhoea (see table 2, p 66). Donepezil was well tolerated in the RCTs. Common adverse effects such as nausea, vomiting, and diarrhoea tended to be mild and transient. Hepatotoxicity was reported as non-significant. All-cause withdrawal reported in systematic review: 27% of people taking 10 mg donepezil, compared with 20% with 5 mg and 21% with placebo.[17] Long term follow up of individuals on donepezil up to 10 mg (open label extension) found 86% experienced at least one adverse effect, often occurring later in the study. Common events included agitation (24%), pain (20%), insomnia (11%), and diarrhoea (9%).[21] We found no evidence of harms specific to populations with vascular or Lewy body dementia.

Comment: Donepezil appears relatively safe and confers some benefit for some individuals. However, pragmatic trials in routine clinical settings are required. Quality of life of carers has not been assessed in existing trials.[17] Donepezil is taken once daily; this is a potential advantage over other cholinesterase inhibitors for people with dementia. Improvement usually starts within 2–4 months of starting donepezil, and onset of improvement is less likely after that time. Open label studies should be interpreted with caution, but do suggest that the effect of continued treatment is sustained in the long term.[21] Many trials that found benefit from donepezil also found much higher withdrawal rates (30% or more) with donepezil than with placebo. In some of these studies, missing data were managed using "last observation carried forward", which does not account for the tendency of people with dementia to deteriorate with time; therefore, these studies may overestimate the benefit derived from donepezil.

OPTION   RIVASTIGMINE

One systematic review has found that rivastigmine improves cognitive function in people with Alzheimer's disease, but adverse effects are common. We found no evidence about the effects of rivastigmine in people with vascular dementia. One RCT in people with Lewy body dementia found improvement of cognitive function and behaviour with rivastigmine versus placebo.

Benefits: **Alzheimer's disease:** We found one systematic review (search date 2000, 4 RCTs, 3370 people with mild to moderate Alzheimer's disease).[18] The review found that over 26 weeks, rivastigmine (6–12 mg) versus placebo produced small but significant improvements in cognitive function (Alzheimer's Disease Assessment Scale cognitive subscale [ADAS-cog]: WMD −2.1, 95% CI −2.7 to −1.5; Mini Mental State Examination: WMD 0.8, 95% CI 0.5 to 1.1), and clinical global state (Clinician's Interview Based Impression of Change: OR 0.7, 95% CI 0.6 to 0.9). Quality of life results were not provided. **Vascular dementia:** We found no systematic review or RCTs of rivastigmine in people with vascular dementia. A subgroup analysis of an RCT (699 people with Alzheimer's disease but not vascular dementia) comparing rivastigmine (1–4 mg daily or 6–12 mg daily) versus placebo over 26 weeks found that people with vascular risk factors responded more than those without (mean ADAS-cog difference −2.3).[22] **Lewy body dementia:** We found no systematic review but found one RCT (120 people with Lewy body dementia), which found that rivastigmine (dose titrated to 6 mg twice daily) versus placebo for 20 weeks significantly improved a computerised psychometric measure of cognitive function (intention to treat analysis; P = 0.05; further exploration of effect size not possible) and a global measure of behavioural function (NNT for at least 30% improvement on Neuropsychiatric Inventory score 3, 95% CI 2 to 6).[23]

Harms: Rivastigmine versus placebo increased the frequency of nausea, vomiting, anorexia, diarrhoea, and discontinuation of treatment (35% with 6–12 mg rivastigmine v 18% with 1–4 mg rivastigmine v 17% with placebo).[18]

Comment: The rates of adverse effects seemed higher with rivastigmine than with other anticholinesterase drugs, but direct comparisons have not been performed.

OPTION   GALANTAMINE

One systematic review has found that galantamine improves cognition and functioning in older people with Alzheimer's disease. We found no evidence about galantamine in people with vascular or Lewy body dementia.

Benefits: **Alzheimer's disease:** We found one systematic review of galantamine versus placebo (search date 2000, 7 RCTs)[19] and one additional RCT (653 people over 26 wks).[24] The systematic review found that galantamine (24 mg twice daily) versus placebo for 6 months improved cognitive function (3 RCTs, 1306 people; Alzheimer's Disease Assessment Scale cognitive subscale [ADAS-cog] score: WMD –3.3, 95% CI –3.9 to –2.7; NNT for 4 point change 7, 95% CI 5 to 12), global status (Clinician's Interview Based Impression of Change: OR 1.8, 95% CI 1.5 to 2.3), and psychiatric symptoms (neuropsychiatric inventory score: WMD –2.3, 95% CI –4.0 to –0.6).[19] Similar results were found with galantamine 32 mg twice daily) versus placebo (2 RCTs, 768 people) (see table 1, p 65). The additional RCT found that galantamine (24 mg daily) versus placebo improved cognitive function (ADAS-cog mean difference: –3.1, 95% CI –4.5 to –1.7).[24] Galantamine (32 mg daily) versus placebo significantly improved cognitive function (ADAS-cog mean difference: –4.1, 95% CI –5.6 to –2.7; NNT for 4 point difference 6, 95% CI 4 to 12) and disability (disability assessment scale, 100 point scale, higher score = better function: mean difference: 3.4, 95% CI 0.1 to 6.7).[24] **Vascular dementia:** We found no systematic review or RCTs of galantamine versus placebo in people with vascular dementia. **Lewy body dementia:** We found no systematic review or RCTs of galantamine versus placebo in people with Lewy body dementia.

Harms: Adverse effects were more frequent with larger doses of galantamine, including nausea (44% with galantamine 13 mg v 13% with placebo), vomiting (20% with galantamine v 8% with placebo), and discontinuation of treatment (38% with galantamine 32 mg daily v 25% with galantamine 24 mg v 16% with placebo).[23]

Comment: None.

OPTION   TACRINE

Two systematic reviews found limited evidence that tacrine improved cognitive function and global state in Alzheimer's disease. We found no evidence about its use in people with vascular or Lewy body dementia. Adverse effects are common.

Dementia

Benefits: **Alzheimer's disease:** We found two systematic reviews of tacrine versus placebo in people with Alzheimer's disease (search date not stated, 12 RCTs, 1984 people;[25] search date 1997, 21 RCTs, 3555 people[26]). Various doses of tacrine were used in the RCTs, and the duration of treatment varied from 3–36 weeks. Tacrine versus placebo significantly improved overall clinical improvement (OR 1.58, 95% CI 1.18 to 2.11), cognition (Mini Mental State Examination at 12 wks: standardised mean differences [SMD] +0.77, 95% CI –0.35 to +1.20; Alzheimer's Disease Assessment Scale cognitive subscale results not provided).[25] A subsequent subgroup analysis indicated that the five non-industry sponsored studies found no significant effect with tacrine versus placebo, but most (6/7) manufacturer supported studies found clinical benefit (1 RCT was not located for the subgroup analysis).[27] **Vascular dementia:** We found no systematic review and no RCTs of tacrine in people with vascular dementia. **Lewy body dementia:** We found no systematic review and no RCTs.

Harms: Withdrawals because of adverse events were common (OR for withdrawal 3.6, 95% CI 2.8 to 4.7)[25] and were more likely with higher doses (265/479 [55%] with high dose tacrine v 20/184 [11%] with placebo), and reversible elevation of liver enzymes was found in 133/265 (50%).[28] Common adverse events included nausea and vomiting (35% with 160 mg daily), diarrhoea (18%), anorexia (12%), and abdominal pain (9%).

Comment: The previous Cochrane review on tacrine has been withdrawn (issue 2, 2001). The quality of tacrine trials was generally poor. The longest RCT lasted 30 weeks.[28] Doses varied considerably among trials. Tacrine has a very high rate of harms.

OPTION	PHYSOSTIGMINE

One systematic review found slow release physostigmine versus placebo in people with Alzheimer's disease improved cognition, but adverse effects were common. We found no evidence about its use in people with vascular or Lewy body dementia.

Benefits: **Alzheimer's disease:** We found one systematic review (search date 2000, 15 RCTs).[29] The RCTs differed widely in the preparations of physostigmine used, which makes it difficult to generalise results. Four RCTs were small trials of intravenous physostigmine, and seven were small trials (131 people) of standard oral preparation. Four RCTs (1456 people) used controlled release preparations. Two RCTs reported results only for people who responded to physostigmine in a prestudy titration phase. One RCT (170 people) found that physostigmine (27 mg daily) versus placebo improved cognition after 12 weeks (Alzheimer's Disease Assessment Scale cognitive subscale: –2.0, 95% CI –3.6 to –0.5), but did not significantly improve activities of daily living or clinician impression of change. **Vascular dementia:** We found no systematic review and no RCTs in people with vascular dementia. **Lewy body dementia:** We found no systematic review and no RCTs.

Harms: Common adverse effects include nausea, vomiting, diarrhoea, dizziness, and stomach pain. In RCTs, that randomised all people with Alzheimer's disease rather than selecting those who tolerated and responded to physostigmine, withdrawals were more common with physostigmine (234/358 [65%] with physostigmine v 31/117 [26%] with placebo; OR 4.80, 95% CI 3.17 to 7.33).[29]

Comment: Physostigmine has a very short half life. We found only limited evidence that physostigmine improved cognition, and no evidence that it improved other domains of function. Adverse affects are common. Screening out non-responders before the trial is likely to overestimate the true effect size.

OPTION   NICOTINE

We found one systematic review, which found no RCTs of adequate quality.

Benefits: One systematic review (search date 2001) found no RCTs of adequate quality.[30]

Harms: We found no RCTs.

Comment: None.

OPTION   LECITHIN

One systematic review in people with Alzheimer's disease found no significant benefit with lecithin versus placebo. We found insufficient evidence about lecithin versus placebo in people with vascular and Lewy body dementia.

Benefits: **Alzheimer's disease:** We found one systematic review (search date 2000, 10 RCTs, 256 people with mild to severe disease Alzheimer's disease) of lecithin, which found no significant improvement in cognition, functional performance, quality of life, or global impression.[31] **Vascular dementia:** We found no systematic review or RCTs. **Lewy body dementia:** We found one systematic review[31] including one RCT (90 people with "Parkinsonian dementia", which may have included people with causes of dementia apart from Lewy body dementia). The RCT found no benefit from lecithin versus placebo.

Harms: The review found that adverse effects were more common with lecithin (41% with lecithin v 10% with placebo; OR 6.0, 95% CI 1.5 to 24).[31] The specific nature of the adverse effects was not stated.

Comment: One RCT (included in the systematic review[31]), of lecithin versus placebo in people with minimal cognitive impairment, found some components of cognition were significantly better in the placebo group. Most studies of lecithin are small and old. Meta-analysis in the systematic review was hampered by diverse outcome criteria. We found no good evidence that lecithin is beneficial in dementia.

OPTION   NON-STEROIDAL ANTI-INFLAMMATORY DRUGS

Two RCTs found conflicting evidence about non-steroidal anti-inflammatory drugs versus placebo in people with Alzheimer's disease. We found no evidence about non-steroidal anti-inflammatory drugs in people with vascular or Lewy body dementia.

Benefits: **Alzheimer's disease:** We found no systematic review but found two RCTs.[32,33] The first RCT (41 people) found that diclofenac plus misoprostol versus placebo for 25 weeks produced no significant difference in cognitive function (Alzheimer's Disease Assessment Scale cognitive subscale [ADAS-cog] score: mean difference +1.14, 95% CI −2.9 to +5.2) or global status (Clinician's Interview Based Impression of Change score: +0.24, 95% CI −0.26 to +0.74).[32] The second RCT (44 people with mild to moderate Alzheimer's disease) found that indomethacin (up to 150 mg daily) versus placebo for 6 months significantly improved cognitive function (Mini Mental State Examination and ADAS; inadequately described results for only 28/44 completers, 14 in each arm).[33] **Vascular dementia:** We found one systematic review of aspirin for vascular dementia (search date 2000) that found no RCTs (see comment below).[34] **Lewy body dementia:** We found no systematic review and no RCTs.

Harms: See non-steroidal anti-inflammatory drugs, p 1063. In one RCT,[32] more people withdrew by week 25 with diclofenac plus misoprostol versus placebo (12 [50%] v 2 [12%]). No serious drug related adverse events were reported.[32] In the RCT of indomethacin, 21% of people on indomethacin withdrew because of gastrointestinal symptoms. [33]

Comment: Earlier versions of a systematic review of aspirin in vascular dementia[34] included one RCT (70 people with vascular dementia), which was subsequently removed because of inadequate quality, including a lack of placebo control.

OPTION   HORMONE REPLACEMENT THERAPY

One systematic review in women with established Alzheimer's disease has found that hormone replacement therapy versus no hormone replacement therapy improves cognition. We found no evidence about its use in people with vascular or Lewy body dementia.

Benefits: **Alzheimer's disease:** We found one systematic review (search date 2000, 8 placebo controlled RCTs of oestrogen 0.625–1.25 mg daily, 313 people, 7 wks to 12 months' duration).[35] The review found that hormone replacement therapy (HRT) versus no HRT improved cognitive function (5 RCTs, Mini Mental State Examination [MMSE]: WMD 2.3, 95% CI 1.7 to 3.4). The largest and longest RCT (120 women with mild to moderate Alzheimer's disease) found that oestrogen (0.625 mg daily) versus placebo for 52 weeks had no significant effect on the Clinical Global Impression of Change 7 point scale, on secondary outcome measures, or on MMSE score at 12 months.[36] **Vascular dementia:** We found no systematic review or RCTs. **Lewy body dementia:** We found no systematic review or RCTs.

Harms: There is concern that oestrogen treatment may increase the risk of developing breast cancer.

Comment: Most RCTs in the meta-analysis were small and heterogeneity may have distorted the results. A meta-analysis of 14 observational studies (5990 people, length of follow up not stated) found that HRT is associated with a lower risk of developing dementia (dementia in 13% with HRT v 21% with controls; RR 0.56, 95% CI 0.46 to 0.68). Observational studies provide only indirect evidence; the observed association may be explained by confounders (e.g. educational level, lifestyle factors).

OPTION   VITAMIN E

One RCT of vitamin E versus placebo in people with Alzheimer's disease found no clear evidence of benefit. We found no evidence about vitamin E in vascular or Lewy body dementia.

Benefits: **Alzheimer's disease:** We found one systematic review (search date 2000, 1 RCT, 169 people with moderate to severe Alzheimer's disease).[37] The multicentre RCT[38] compared high dose α-tocopherol (vitamin E, 2000 IU daily) versus placebo and compared selegiline versus placebo. It found that high dose α-tocopherol versus placebo for 2 years did not significantly affect cognitive function (measured by the cognitive portion of the Alzheimer's Disease Assessment Scale). Those taking vitamin E were less likely to reach one of four predefined end points: death, institutionalisation, loss of ability to perform activities of daily living, or decrease in global rating (combined OR 0.49, 95% CI 0.25 to 0.96). **Vascular dementia:** We found no systematic review or RCTs. **Lewy body dementia:** We found no systematic review or RCTs.

Harms: The RCT found no significant differences in adverse effects between placebo and α-tocopherol.[38] Other studies have found weak evidence of associations between high dose α-tocopherol and bowel irritation, headache, muscular weakness, visual complaints, vaginal bleeding, bruising, thrombophlebitis, deterioration of angina pectoris, worsening of diabetes, syncope, and dizziness.[39] A few case reports have created concern that vitamin E may increase the risk of haemorrhagic stroke.

Comment: The groups in the RCT[38] were not matched evenly at baseline: the placebo group had a higher mean Mini Mental State Examination score, and these baseline scores were a significant predictor of outcome. Attempts to correct for this imbalance suggested that α-tocopherol might increase mean survival, but the need for statistical adjustments weakens the strength of this conclusion.

OPTION   SELEGILINE

One systematic review has found that in people with Alzheimer's disease, selegiline versus placebo improves cognitive function, behavioural disturbance, and mood, but found no evidence of improved clinical global state. Selegiline was well tolerated and no serious adverse events were reported. We found no evidence about its use in vascular or Lewy body dementia.

Benefits: **Alzheimer's disease:** We found one systematic review (search date not stated, 15 RCTs)[40] comparing selegiline versus placebo (average number of people 50, typical duration of treatment 3 months). Analysis of pooled results found that selegiline improved several outcome measures: cognitive function scores (measured by several parameters: SMD –0.56, 95% CI –0.88 to –0.24), mood score (Dementia Mood Assessment Scale: SMD –1.14, 95% CI –2.11 to –0.18), and behavioural symptom score (Brief Psychiatric Rating Scale: SMD –0.53, 95% CI –0.94 to –0.12). The review found no evidence of an effect on global rating scales (SMD –0.11, 95% CI –0.49 to +0.27). **Vascular dementia:** We found no systematic review or RCTs. **Lewy body dementia:** We found no systematic review or RCTs.

Harms: Withdrawal rates were low (14/15 [93%]) and most studies found no significant difference between groups.[41] The RCTs reported no major adverse events.

Comment: The trials used a variety of outcomes, making comparison with other treatments difficult.

OPTION	GINKGO BILOBA

One systematic review has found good evidence that Ginkgo biloba versus placebo improves cognitive function and is well tolerated in Alzheimer's disease. We found no clear evidence to support its use in vascular or Lewy body dementia.

Benefits: **Alzheimer's disease:** We found one systematic review[42] and one subsequent RCT.[43] The systematic review (search date 1998, 9 double blind RCTs in people with Alzheimer's disease, vascular dementia, or mixed Alzheimer's disease/vascular dementia)[42] found that in eight RCTs Ginkgo biloba was superior to placebo for a variety of outcomes. The largest and longest trial (52 wks, 309 people of which 236 had Alzheimer's disease) found that in people with Alzheimer's disease, Ginkgo biloba versus placebo significantly improved cognition (completer analysis for people with Alzheimer's disease or vascular dementia, change in Alzheimer's Disease Assessment Scale cognitive subscale [ADAS-cog] score: –1.7, 95% CI –3.2 to –0.20; NNT for 4 point change in ADAS-cog: 8, 95% CI 5 to 50), care giver assessed improvement (change in Geriatric Evaluation by Relative's Rating Instrument score: –0.19, 95% CI –0.28 to –0.08), but did not significantly improve the mean Clinician's Global Impression of Change score (change in score: 0, 95% CI –0.2 to +0.2).[44] The RCT had a high withdrawal rate (137 people [44%] withdrew). The subsequent RCT (24 wks, 214 people in elderly people homes) compared Ginkgo biloba 240 mg daily versus Ginkgo biloba 160 mg daily versus placebo in people with dementia (30%) or mild cognitive impairment (70%).[43] People receiving active medication were re-randomised after 12 weeks to continuing active medication or placebo. Placebo included quinine to mimic the bitter taste of Ginkgo biloba. The study found no significant benefits for Ginkgo biloba. **Vascular dementia:** One systematic review[42] included a meta-analysis for people with vascular dementia, and one subsequent RCT[43] separately analysed results for people with vascular dementia. No benefits were found for Ginkgo biloba versus placebo. **Lewy body dementia:** We found no systematic review or RCTs.

Harms: The largest RCT found adverse events were equally likely with Ginkgo biloba versus placebo (31% v 31%).[44] No specific pattern of adverse events was reported.

Comment: Most of the RCTs were brief, with different entry criteria, outcomes, and doses. The effect size of Ginkgo biloba was minimal in the study that used a bitter tasting placebo.[43] De-blinding is common in dementia trials, and may account for some of the perceived treatment effect. However, 70% of the people in this study did not meet criteria for dementia, so the true effect size is uncertain. The high withdrawal rate in the largest RCT weakens its conclusions, although the authors did conduct both completer and intention to treat analyses.[44]

OPTION   REMINISCENCE THERAPY

We found insufficient evidence on the effects of reminiscence therapy in people with unspecified dementia.

Benefits: We found one systematic review of reminiscence therapy (see glossary, p 61) (search date 1998, 2 RCTs).[45] Analysis of pooled data was hindered by poor trial methods, diverse outcomes, and no separation of data for different types of dementia.

Harms: We found no evidence.

Comment: None.

OPTION   REALITY ORIENTATION

One systematic review found that reality orientation improved cognitive function and behaviour compared with no treatment in people with unspecified dementia. We found no evidence about harms.

Benefits: We found one systematic review (search date 1997, 6 RCTs, 125 people).[46] The RCTs compared reality orientation (see glossary, p 61) versus no treatment and used different measures of cognition. The review found that reality orientation improved cognitive function score (SMD −0.59, 95% CI −0.95 to −0.22) and behavioural symptom score (SMD −0.66, 95% CI −1.27 to −0.05). No separate analysis was done for specific types of dementia.

Harms: The RCTs gave no information on adverse effects.[46]

Comment: The RCTs did not use standardised interventions or outcomes.[46]

OPTION   MUSIC THERAPY

One systematic review of numerous studies with weak methods found insufficient evidence about music therapy.

Benefits: We found one systematic review of music therapy (search date 1998, 21 studies, 336 people).[47] It included studies with weak methods and found in a meta-analysis that music therapy versus control interventions significantly improved reported outcomes (mean effect size 0.79, 95% CI 0.62 to 0.95). Significant effects were noted with different types of music therapy (active v passive, taped v live).

Harms: Harms were not stated.

Comment: The primary studies lacked adequate controls, had potential for bias, used diverse interventions, and used inadequate outcome measures. Although one meta-analysis found significant benefits for music therapy on pooling the results of many studies, further high quality studies are needed to clarify whether the results are explained by a true effect or by bias. A previous Cochrane systematic review has been withdrawn.[48]

QUESTION **What are the effects of treatments on behavioural and psychological symptoms of dementia?**

OPTION **ANTIPSYCHOTICS**

One systematic review has found that antipsychotics versus placebo produce a small but significant improvement of behavioural disorders in people with unspecified dementia. Three subsequent RCTs have found that risperidone, and olanzapine reduce behavioural problems or psychosis, wheras two RCTs have found no significant improvement with haloperidol compared with placebo.

Benefits: We found one systematic review (search date 1995, 16 RCTs, 4–12 wks' duration, 734 people with unspecified dementia and behavioural problems).[49] It found that antipsychotics versus placebo increased the number of people who improved (64%, 95% CI 54% to 74% with antipsychotic v 34%, 95% CI 18% to 50% with placebo). The most commonly used antipsychotics were haloperidol (8 RCTs) and thioridazine (6 RCTs). The review found no difference in efficacy between different antipsychotic groups. **Comparisons between antipsychotics:** One RCT (344 people with severe dementia, mean age 81 years, 56% women) compared adjusted doses of risperidone (mean dose 1.1 mg, 115 people) versus haloperidol (mean dose 1.2 mg, 115 people) versus placebo (114 people) over 13 weeks for the treatment of behavioural symptoms.[50] A response was defined as a reduction of at least 30% in the Behave-AD scale. Risperidone had no significant effect on the number of responders compared with placebo (37/68 [54%] with risperidone v 35/74 [47%] with placebo; ARI +7%, 95% CI, −9% to +23%). Haloperidol increased the number of responders compared with placebo (51/81 [63%] with haloperidol; ARI 15%, 95% CI 0% to 31%; P = 0.05), but the difference between risperidone and haloperidol was not significant. **Risperidone:** One RCT (double blind, 625 people with moderate to severe dementia plus behavioural and psychological symptoms, 73% with Alzheimer's disease, mean age 83 years, 68% women) compared risperidone versus placebo over 12 weeks.[51] A response was defined as a reduction of at least 50% in the Behave-AD scale. Compared with placebo, risperidone 1 and 2 mg significantly improved the chance of responding (45% with risperidone 1 mg v 33% with placebo v 50% with risperidone 2 mg; for risperidone 1 mg v placebo NNT 9, 95% CI 5 to 100; for risperidone 2 mg v placebo NNT 6, 95% CI 4 to 17). Gender and the type of dementia did not significantly affect the results. **Olanzapine:** We found one RCT (double blind, 6 wks' duration, 206 elderly US nursing home residents with Alzheimer's disease plus psychotic or behavioural symptoms).[52] The RCT compared olanzapine (given as a fixed dose of 5, 10, or 15 mg daily) versus placebo. Agitation, hallucinations, and delusions were improved by the two lower doses but not by the highest dose of olanzapine when compared with placebo (subscale of the neuropsychiatric inventory [nursing home version]: −7.6 with olanzapine 5 mg v −6.1 with olanzapine 10 mg v −4.9 with olanzapine 15 mg v −3.7 with placebo). **Haloperidol:** We found two RCTs, which found no significant improvement with haloperidol versus placebo.[53,54] The first RCT (double blind, 6 wks' duration, 71 outpatients with Alzheimer's disease) compared standard dose haloperidol (2–3 mg daily) versus low dose haloperidol (0.5–0.75 mg daily) versus placebo for the treatment of psychosis and disruptive behaviours.[53] It found no significant difference in the number of responders (reduction of 25% or more on the Brief Psychiatric Rating Scale psychosis factor score: 12/20 [60%] with standard dose haloperidol v 6/20 [30%] with low dose haloperidol v 6/20 [30%] placebo; overall P < 0.06). The second RCT (double blind, 149 people with Alzheimer's disease, 16 wks' duration) found no significant differences in the reduction of agitation (main outcome was the Alzheimer's Disease Co-operative Study Clinical Global Impression of Change score) between the four interventions (haloperidol 1.1 mg daily v trazodone 200 mg daily v behaviour management techniques v placebo).[54]

Harms: In the systematic review, adverse effects were more common with antipsychotics than placebo (ARI 25%, 95% CI 13% to 37%), including sedation (21%), movement disorders (13%), and orthostatic hypotension (8%). However, pooled withdrawal rates were not different between antipsychotics and placebo (ARI 4%, 95% CI −7% to 14%). The first RCT of risperidone found discontinuation because of adverse events was more common with high dose risperidone (12% with placebo v 8% with 0.5 mg v 16% with 1 mg v 24% with 2 mg) but in the second RCT about 18% of people withdrew because of adverse effects from each of the three arms. With olanzapine, increased adverse effects were sedation (6% with placebo v 25% with 5 mg v 26% with 10 mg v 36% with 15 mg), and gait disturbance (2% with placebo v 20% with 5 mg v 14% with 10 mg v 17% with 15 mg). Extrapyramidal adverse effects were more common in people receiving haloperidol than placebo (22% with haloperidol v 15% with risperidone v 11% with placebo). One study (2 year prospective, longitudinal, 71 people with dementia) found that the mean decline in cognitive scores in 16 people who took antipsychotics was twice that of people who did not (expanded Mini Mental State Examination 21 v 9; P = 0.002). See schizophrenia, p 920.[55]

Comment: Most studies suggest that antipsychotic medications are effective at reducing behavioural and psychiatric symptoms in people with dementia. However, high response rates with placebo indicate that many behavioural problems resolve spontaneously in the short term. Most people with dementia are sensitive to adverse effects from antipsychotics, especially sedation and extrapyramidal symptoms. People with Lewy body dementia are particularly sensitive to these adverse effects, suggesting that antipsychotics have a poor balance of benefits and harms in people with Lewy body dementia. More studies are needed to determine whether newer atypical antipsychotics have a better ratio of benefits to harms than older antipsychotics.

OPTION   ANTIEPILEPTIC DRUGS

One RCT found that carbamazepine versus placebo reduced agitation and aggression in people with unspecified dementia. Another RCT found that sodium valproate reduced agitation in unspecified dementia. We found no evidence about other antiepileptic drugs.

Benefits: We found no systematic review but we found two RCTs.[56,57] The first RCT (semi-blind, 51 nursing home patients with agitation and dementia, 6 wks' duration) compared carbamazepine (individualised doses; modal dose 300 mg; mean serum level 5.3 µg/mL versus placebo).[56] It found that carbamazepine versus placebo significantly improved a measure of agitation and aggression (mean total Brief Psychiatric Rating Scale [BPRS] score: 7.7 with carbamazepine v 0.9 with placebo) and a measure of global status (Clinical Global Impressions [CGI] rating: 77% with carbamazepine v 21% with placebo). The second RCT (semi-blind, 56 people in nursing homes, 6 wks' duration) compared sodium valproate with placebo.[57] It found that when several covariates were taken into account, sodium valproate improved agitation and aggression (measured by BPRS score; $P = 0.05$ only after adjustment), and a measure of global status (CGI rating: 68% with sodium valproate v 52% with placebo; $P = 0.06$).

Harms: Harms were significantly more common with carbamazepine than with placebo (16/27 [59%] v 7/24 [29%]; $P = 0.003$). These were considered clinically significant in two cases (1 person with tics, 1 with ataxia). Carbamazepine in the elderly may cause cardiac toxicity. Harms, which were generally rated as mild, were also more common with sodium valproate than with placebo (68% sodium valproate v 33% with placebo; $P = 0.003$).[57]

Comment: The need to perform adjustments for covariates in the second RCT weakens the strength of the findings.

OPTION   ANTIDEPRESSANTS

One RCT in people with dementia plus agitated behaviour found no significant difference in benefits between trazodone versus haloperidol. Another RCT found no significant difference between trazodone versus placebo.

Benefits: **Trazodone:** We found no systematic review but found two RCTs. The first small RCT (double blind, 28 elderly people with dementia and agitated behaviour, 9 wks' duration) compared trazodone (50–250 mg daily) versus haloperidol (1–5 mg daily).[58] It found no significant difference in agitation between the groups, but the trial was too small to exclude a clinically important difference. The second RCT (double blind, 149 people with Alzheimer's disease, 16 wks' duration) compared the reduction of agitation with haloperidol (mean dose 1.1 mg daily) versus trazodone (mean dose 200 mg daily) versus behaviour management techniques versus placebo.[54]

It found no significant differences in outcome (Alzheimer's Disease Co-operative Study Clinical Global Impression of Change) between the four interventions.

Harms: In the first RCT[58] adverse effects were more common in the group treated with haloperidol than trazodone. In the second RCT no significant differences in adverse events were seen between the trazodone group and the placebo group.[54] Priapism has been reported with trazodone, occurring in about 1/10 000 people.

Comment: The RCTs were too small to exclude clinically important differences between the interventions.

OPTION	BEHAVIOUR MANAGEMENT

Three RCTs have compared behaviour management versus control treatments as treatment of behaviour disorders in people with non-specified dementia. The RCTs used different behavioural interventions but each included components of expert analysis of behavioural problems plus education of carers. One study found a significant reduction in behavioural disorders but the other two RCTs found benefits that were not significant.

Benefits: We found no systematic review but found three RCTs.[54,59,60] One RCT (81 people with dementia and behaviour disorders in nursing homes) found that a dementia care programme (consisting of activities, guidelines for psychotropic medications, and 1 h of education/wk) versus usual nursing home care reduced the number of people with behaviour disorders (12/42 [29%] v 20/39 [51%]; OR 0.4, 95% CI 0.2 to 1.0).[59] Controls were more likely to receive antipsychotics (OR 2.6, 95% CI 1.0 to 6.8; P = 0.06). The second RCT (62 people with dementia, 10 wks' duration) found that, over 8 weeks, four sessions of a community based behaviour management programme versus usual care non-significantly reduced aggressive behaviour (rating scale for aggressive behaviour in the elderly: from 9.4 – 6.9 with behaviour management v from 8.8 – 8.6 with control).[60] The third RCT (double blind, 149 people with Alzheimer's disease, 16 wks' duration) compared the effects on agitation of haloperidol (mean dose 1.1 mg daily) versus trazodone (mean dose 200 mg daily) versus behaviour management techniques versus placebo.[54] It found no significant differences in outcome (Alzheimer's Disease Co-operative Study Clinical Global Impression of Change) between the four interventions.

Harms: No harms were identified with behaviour management.

Comment: None.

GLOSSARY

Reality orientation Involves presenting information that is designed to reorient a person in time, place, or person. It may range in intensity from a board giving details of the day, date, and season, to staff reorienting a patient at each contact.

Reminiscence therapy Involves encouraging people to talk about the past in order to enable past experiences to be brought into consciousness. It relies on remote memory, which is relatively well preserved in mild to moderate dementia.

Dementia

REFERENCES

1. van Duijn CM. Epidemiology of the dementia: recent developments and new approaches *J Neurol Neurosurg Psychiatry* 1996;60:478–488.
2. McKeith IG, Galasko D, Kosaka K, et al. Consensus guidelines for the clinical and pathological diagnosis of dementia with Lewy bodies (DLB): report of the consortium on DLB International workshop. *Neurology* 1996;47:1113–1124.
3. Rasmusson DX, Brandt J, Steele C, Hedreen JC, Troncoso JC, Folstein MF. Accuracy of clinical diagnosis of Alzheimer disease and clinical features of patients with non-Alzheimer's disease neuropathology. *Alzheimer Dis Assoc Disord* 1996; 10:180–188.
4. Verghese J, Crystal HA, Dickson DW, Lipton RB. Validity of clinical criteria for the diagnosis of dementia with Lewy bodies. *Neurology* 1999;53: 1974–1982.
5. Lobo A, Launer LJ, Fratiglioni L, et al. Prevalence of dementia and major subtypes in Europe: a collaborative study of population-based cohorts. *Neurology* 2000;54:S4–S9.
6. Farrer L. Intercontinental epidemiology of Alzheimer's disease: a global approach to bad gene hunting. *JAMA* 2001;285:796–798.
7. Skoog I. A population-based study of dementia in 85 year olds. *N Engl J Med* 1993;328:153–158.
8. McKeith IG. Clinical Lewy body syndromes. *Ann N Y Acad Sci* 2000;920:1–8.
9. Inkeda M, Hokoishi K, Maki N, et al. Increased prevalence of vascular dementia in Japan: a community-based epidemiological study. *Neurology* 2001;57:839–844.
10. McKeith I. The differential diagnosis of dementia. In: Burns A, Levy R, eds. *Dementia*. 1st ed. London: Chapman and Hall, 1994:39–57.
11. Hardy J. Molecular classification of Alzheimer's disease. *Lancet* 1991;1:1342–1343.
12. Eastwood R, Reisberg B. Mood and behaviour. In: Panisset M, Stern Y, Gauthier S, eds. *Clinical diagnosis and management of Alzheimer's disease*. 1st ed. London: Dunitz, 1996:175–189.
13. Absher JR, Cummings JL. Cognitive and noncognitive aspects of dementia syndromes. In: Burns A, Levy R, eds. *Dementia*. 1st ed. London: Chapman and Hall, 1994:59–76.
14. Rosen WG, Mohs RC, Davis KL. A new rating scale for Alzheimer's disease. *Am J Psychiatry* 1984; 141:1356–1364.
15. Folstein MF, Folstein SE, McHugh PR. Mini Mental State: a practical method for grading the cognitive state of patients for the clinician. *J Psychiatr Res* 1975;12:189–198.
16. Burns A, Lawlor B, Craig S. Assessment scales in old age psychiatry. London: Martin Dunitz.1998
17. Birks JS, Melzer D, Beppu H. Donepezil for mild and moderate Alzheimer's disease (Cochrane Review). In: The Cochrane Library, Issue 1, 2001. Oxford: Update Software. Search date 2000; primary sources Cochrane Dementia and Cognitive Impairment Group Specialized Register of Clinical Trials, Medline, Psychlit, Embase, the Donepezil Study Group, and Eisai Inc.
18. Birks J, Iakovidou V, Tsolaki M, et al. Rivastigmine for Alzheimer's disease (Cochrane Review). In: The Cochrane Library, Issue 1, 2001. Oxford: Update Software. Search date 2000; primary sources Cochrane Controlled Trials Register, Cochrane Dementia Group Specialized Register of Clinical Trials, Medline, Embase, Psychlit, Cinahl, and hand searches of geriatric and dementia journals and conference abstracts.
19. Olin J, Schneider L. Galantamine for Alzheimer's disease (Cochrane review). In: The Cochrane Library, Issue 1, 2001. Oxford: Update Software. Search date 2000; primary sources Cochrane Dementia Group Specialized Register of Clinical Trials, Cochrane Controlled Trials Register, Embase, Medline, Psychlit, Combined Health Information Database, National Research Register, Alzheimer's Disease Education and Referral Centre Clinical Database, Biomed (Biomedicine and Health), GlaxoWellcome Clinical Trials Register, National Institutes of Health Clinical Trials Databases, Current Controlled Trials, Dissertation Abstracts, Index to UK Theses, hand searched reference lists, and additional information was collected from an unpublished investigational brochure for galantamine.
20. Rogers SL, Farlow MR, Doody RS, Mohs R, Friedhoff LT. A 24-week double blind placebo controlled trial of donepezil in patients with Alzheimer's disease. *Neurology* 1998;50: 136–145.
21. Rogers SL, Doody RS, Pratt RD, Ieni JR. Long term efficacy and safety of donepezil in the treatment of Alzheimer's disease: final analysis of a US multicentre open-label study. Eur *Neuropsychopharmacol* 2000;10:195–203.
22. Kumar V, Anand R, Messina J, et al. An efficacy and safety analysis of Exelon in Alzheimer's disease patients with concurrent vascular risk factors. *Eur J Neurol* 2000;7:159–169.
23. McKeith I, Del Ser T, Spano P, et al. Efficacy of rivastigmine in dementia with Lewy bodies: a randomised, double-blind, placebo-controlled international study. *Lancet* 2000;356: 2031–2036.
24. Wilcock G, Lilienfield S, Gaens E. Efficacy and safety of galantamine in patients with mild to moderate Alzheimer's disease: multicentre randomised controlled trial. *BMJ* 2000;321:1–7.
25. Qizilbash N, Whitehead A, Higgins J, Wilcock G, Schneider L, Farlow M. Cholinesterase inhibition for Alzheimer disease. *JAMA* 1998;280: 1777–1782. Search date not stated; primary sources Cochrane Dementia Group Registry of Clinical Trials, trial investigators, and Park-Davis Pharmaceuticals.
26. Arrieta JR, Artalejo FR. Methodology, results and quality of clinical trials of tacrine in the treatment of Alzheimer's disease: a systematic review of the literature. *Age ageing*.1998;27:161–179. Search date 1997; primary sources Cochrane Library and Medline.
27. Koepp R, Miles SH. Meta-analysis of tacrine for Alzheimer's disease: the influence of industry sponsors. *JAMA* 1999;281:2287–2288.
28. Knapp MJ, Knopman DS, Solomon PR, Pendlebury WW, Davis CS, Gracon SI. A 30-week randomized controlled trial of high-dose tacrine in patients with Alzheimer's disease. The Tacrine Study Group. *JAMA* 1994;271:985–991.
29. Coelho F, Filho JM, Birks J. Physostigmine for Alzheimer's disease (Cochrane Review). In: The Cochrane Library, Issue 3, 2001. Oxford: Update Software. Search date 2000; primary sources the Cochrane Dementia Group Specialized Register of Clinical Trials and pharmaceutical companies.
30. López-Arrieta JM, Rodríguez JL, Sanz F. Efficacy and safety of nicotine on Alzheimer's disease patients (Cochrane Review). In: The Cochrane Library, Issue 3, 2001. Oxford: Update Software. Search date 2001; primary source Cochrane Dementia Group Specialized Register of Clinical Trials.
31. Higgins JPT, Flicker L. Lecithin for dementia and cognitive impairment (Cochrane Review). In: The

Cochrane Library, Issue 3, 2001. Oxford: Update Software. Search date 2000; primary sources Cochrane Dementia and Cognitive Impairment Group Specialized Register of Clinical Trials, Medline, Embase, Psychlit, ISI, Current Contents, and hand searched reference lists and textbooks.

32. Scharf S, Mander A, Ugoni A, Vajda F, Christophidis N. A double-blind, placebo-controlled trial of diclofenac/misoprostol in Alzheimer's disease. *Neurology* 1999;53:197–201.

33. Rogers J, Kirby LC, Hempleman SR, et al. Clinical trial of indomethacin in Alzheimer's disease. *Neurology* 1993;43:1609–1611.

34. Williams PS, Spector A, Orrell M, Rands G. Aspirin for vascular dementia. In: The Cochrane Library, Issue 1, 2001. Oxford: Update Software. Search date 2000; primary sources Medline, Cochrane Library Trials Register, Embase, Cinahl, Psychlit, Amed, Sigle, National Research Register, hand searched reference lists, and contact with specialists.

35. Hogervorst E, Williams J, Budge M, Riedel W, Jolles J. The nature of the effect of female gonadal hormone replacement therapy on cognitive function in post-menopausal women: a meta-analysis. *Neuroscience* 2000;101:485–512. Search date 2000, primary sources Medline, Embase, Psychlit, and hand searches of reference lists.

36. Mulnard RA, Cotman CW, Kawas C, et al. Estrogen replacement therapy for treatment of mild to moderate Alzheimer disease: a randomized controlled trial. Alzheimer's Disease Co-operative Study. *JAMA* 2000;283:1007–1015.

37. Tabet N, Birks J, Grimley Evans J. Vitamin E for Alzheimer's disease (Cochrane review). In: The Cochrane Library, Issue 1, 2001. Oxford: Update Software. Search date 2000; primary sources Cochrane Dementia and Cognitive Impairment Group Specialized Register of Clinical Trials

38. Sano M, Ernesto C, Thomas RG, et al. A controlled trial of selegiline, α-tocopherol, or both as treatment for Alzheimer's disease. *N Engl J Med* 1997;336:1216–1222.

39. Myers DG, Maloley PA, Weeks D. Safety of antioxidant vitamins. *Arch Intern Med* 1996;156:925–935.

40. Birks J, Flicker L. Selegiline for Alzheimer's disease (Cochrane Review). In: The Cochrane Library, Issue 3, 2001. Oxford: Update Software. Search date not stated, review amended 1998; primary source Cochrane Dementia and Cognitive Impairment Group Register of Clinical Trials.

41. Freedman M, Rewilak D, Xerri T, et al. L-deprenyl in Alzheimer's disease. Cognitive and behavioural effects. *Neurology* 1998;50:660–668.

42. Ernst E, Pittler MH. Ginkgo biloba for dementia. *Clin Drug Invest* 1999;17:301–308. Search date 1998; primary sources Medline, Embase, Biosis, Cochrane Register of Controlled Clinical Trials, hand searches of bibliographies, and contact with manufacturers.

43. Van Dongen MC, van Rossum E, Kessels AG, Sielhorst HJ, Knipschild PG. The efficacy of Ginkgo for elderly people with dementia and age-associated memory impairment: New results of a randomised controlled trial. *J Am Geriatr Soc* 2000;48:1183–1194.

44. Le Bars P, Katz MM, Berman N, Itil T, Freedman A, Schatzberg AF. A placebo-controlled, double-blind, randomised trial of an extract of Ginkgo biloba for dementia. *JAMA* 1997;278:1327–1332.

45. Spector A, Orrell M. Reminiscence therapy for dementia. In: The Cochrane Library, Issue 1, 2001. Oxford: Update Software. Search date 1998; primary sources Cochrane Controlled Trials Register, Medline, Psychlit, Embase, Omni, Bids, Dissertation Abstracts International,

Sigle, reference lists of relevant articles, internet sites, and hand searching of specialist journals.

46. Spector A, Orrell M, Davies S, et al. Reality orientation for dementia. In: The Cochrane Library, Issue 1, 2001. Oxford: Update Software. Search date 1997; primary sources Medline, Psychlit, Embase, Cochrane Database of Systematic Reviews, Omni, Bids, Dissertation Abstracts International, Sigle, plus internet searching of HealthWeb, Mental Health Infosources, American Psychiatric Association, Internet Mental Health, Mental Health Net, NHS Confederation, and hand searching of specialist journals.

47. Koger SM, Chaplin K, Brotons M. Is music therapy an effective intervention for dementia? A meta-analytic review of the literature. *J Music Ther* 1999;36:2–15. Search date 1998; primary sources Medline, Psychlit, and hand searched reference lists.

48. Koger SM, Brotons M. Music therapy for dementia symptoms. In: Cochrane Library, Issue 3, 2000. Oxford: Update Software. Search date 2000; primary sources Medline, Cochrane Dementia and Cognitive Improvement Group Trials Register, Embase, Cinahl, and Psychlit.

49. Lanctot KL, Best TS, Mittmann N, et al. Efficacy and safety of neuroleptics in behavioural disorders associated with dementia. *J Clin Psychiatry* 1998;59:550–561. Search date 1995; primary sources Medline and hand search of references.

50. De Deyn PP, Rabheru K, Rasmussen A, et al. A randomized trial of risperidone, placebo, and haloperidol for behavioural symptoms of dementia. *Neurology* 1999;53:946–955.

51. Katz IR, Jeste DV, Mintzer JE, Clyde C, Napolitano J, Brecher M. Comparison of risperidone and placebo for psychosis and behavioural disturbances associated with dementia: a randomized double-blind trial. *J Clin Psychiatry* 1999;60:107–115.

52. Street JS, Clark WS, Gannon KS, et al. Olanzapine treatment of psychotic and behavioural symptoms in patients with Alzheimer's disease in nursing care facilities: a double-blind, randomized, placebo-controlled trial. *Arch Gen Psychiatry* 2000;57:968–976.

53. Devanand DP, Marder K, Michaels KS, et al. A randomised, placebo-controlled dose-comparison trial of haloperidol for psychosis and disruptive behaviours in Alzheimer's disease. *Am J Psychiatry* 1998;155:1512–1520.

54. Teri L, Logsdon RG, Peskind E, et al. Treatment of agitation in AD: a randomised, placebo-controlled clinical trial. *Neurology* 2000;55:1271–1278.

55. McShane R, Keene J, Gedling K, Fairburn C, Jacob R, Hope T. Do neuroleptic drugs hasten cognitive decline in dementia? Prospective study with necropsy follow up. *BMJ* 1997;314:266–269.

56. Tariot PN, Erb R, Podgorski CA, et al. Efficacy and tolerability of carbamazepine for agitation and aggression in dementia. *Am J Psychiatry* 1998;155:54–61.

57. Porsteinsson AOP, Tariot PN, Erb R, et al. Placebo-controlled study of divalproex sodium for agitation in dementia. *Am J Geriatr Psychiatry* 2001;9:58–66.

58. Sultzer DL, Gray KF, Gunay I, Berisford MA, Mahler ME. A double-blind comparison of trazodone and haloperidol for treatment of agitation in patients with dementia. *Am J Geriatr Psychiatry* 1997;5:60–69.

59. Rovner BW, Steele CD, Shmuely DSW, Folstein MF. A randomised trial of dementia care in nursing homes. *J Am Geriatr Soc* 1996;44:7–13.

60. Gormley N, Lyons D, Howard R. Behavioural management of aggression in dementia: a randomised controlled trial. *Age Ageing* 2001;30:141–145.

Dementia

James Warner
Senior Lecturer/Consultant in Old Age
Psychiatry
St Margaret's Hospital
Epping
UK

Rob Butler
Consultant in Old Age Psychiatry
Imperial College of Science Technology
and Medicine
London
UK

Competing interests: JW has been reimbursed by
Novartis, the manufacturer of rivastigmine, for conference
attendance and has received speaker fees from Janssen
Pharmaceuticals for educational events. RB, none
declared.

TABLE 1 Effects of donepezil, rivastigmine, and galantamine on Alzheimer's Disease Assessment Scale cognitive subscale (ADAS-cog) scores (see text, p 49).

Drug	Dose (mg)	Duration (wk)	Number randomised	Effect size (difference in ADAS-cog between treatment and placebo arms) (95% CI)	NNT (95% CI) 4 point change in ADAS-cog	OR (95% CI) for treatment withdrawal	Ref
Donepezil	5	12	488	−2.3 (−3.2 to −1.5)	N/A	2.3 (1.0 to 5.3)	17
		24	831	−1.9 (−2.6 to −1.1)	N/A	0.9 (0.5 to 1.4)	17
	10	12	253	−3.1 (−4.2 to −1.9)	N/A	4.1 (1.6 to 10.4)	17
		24	821	−2.9 (−3.7 to −2.2)	4 (3 to 7)	1.6 (1.1 to 2.3)	17
Rivastigmine	1–4	12	1293	−0.3 (−0.9 to +0.3)	+50 (+25 to −50)	2.7 (1.1 to 6.8)	18
		26	1293	−0.8 (−15 to −0.2)	+100 (+15 to −20)	1.0 (0.7 to 1.5)	18
	6–12	12	1917	−1.5 (−2.0 to −1.0)	15 (10 to 25)	3.1 (1.3 to 7.6)	18
		26	1917	−2.1 (−2.7 to −1.5)	17 (12 to 34)	3.0 (2.3 to 3.8)	18
Galantamine	16	20	565	−3.3 (−4.5 to −2.2)	7 (5 to 13)	1.0 (0.51 to 1.9)	19
	24	20	1352	−3.3 (−3.9 to −2.7)	7 (5 to 12)	1.5 (0.8 to 2.6)	19
	32	24	825	−3.3 (−4.1 to −2.4)	5 (4 to 10)	4.7 (2.9 to 7.5)	19

N/A, not available; ref, reference.

TABLE 2 Common adverse effects of cholinesterase inhibitors (see text, p 49).

	Nausea		Vomiting		Diarrhoea	
	Percentage in treatment group	OR	Percentage in treatment group	OR	Percentage in treatment group	OR
Donepezil 10 mg od	19	3.6 (2.1 to 6.4)	14	2.8 (1.8 to 4.2)	16	2.9 (2.0 to 4.2)
Rivastigmine 6–12 mg bd	47	5.4 (4.4 to 6.6)	31	5.3 (4.2 to 6.7)	19	1.7 (1.4 to 2.3)
Galantamine 24 mg bd	30	3.7 (2.8 to 4.8)	16	3.0 (2.1 to 4.2)	8	1.4 (0.9 to 2.1)

bd, twice daily; od, once daily.

QUESTIONS

INTERVENTIONS

Key Messages

- One systematic review found no evidence of benefit from tricyclic antidepressants in prepubertal children and no clear benefit in adolescents. We found limited evidence on the use of fluoxetine and no evidence to support the use of other serotonin reuptake inhibitor drugs. We found limited evidence to support the use of the reversible monoamine oxidase inhibitor moclobemide, and no evidence to support the use of the non-reversible monoamine oxidase inhibitors, venlafaxine or lithium.
- We found insufficient evidence on the effects of St John's Wort (*Hypericum perforatum*) in children and adolescents with depression.
- We found insufficient evidence on the use of electroconvulsive therapy in children and adolescents with depression.
- One systematic review has found cognitive behavioural therapy to be superior to non-specific supportive therapies for mild to moderate depression in children and adolescents. Two RCTs of interpersonal therapy also suggested benefit compared with no treatment. We found insufficient evidence to conclude that family therapy or group treatments other than cognitive behavioural therapy are effective treatments for depression in children and adolescents. We found no systematic reviews or RCTs looking at long term outcomes for psychological or pharmacological treatments.

DEFINITION See depressive disorders, p 74. Compared with adult depression, depression in children and adolescents may have a more insidious onset, may be characterised more by irritability than sadness, and occurs more often in association with other conditions such as anxiety, conduct disorder, hyperkinesis, and learning problems.[1]

INCIDENCE/ PREVALENCE Estimates of prevalence of depression among children and adolescents in the community range from 2–6%.[2,3] Prevalence tends to increase with age, with a sharp rise around onset of puberty. Pre-adolescent boys and girls are affected equally by the condition, but depression is seen more frequently among adolescent girls than boys.[4]

AETIOLOGY/ RISK FACTORS Uncertain, but may include childhood events and current psychosocial adversity.

PROGNOSIS See prognosis under depressive disorders, p 75. In children and adolescents, the recurrence rate of depressive episodes first occurring in childhood or adolescence is 70% by 5 years, which is similar to the recurrence rate in adults.[5] Young people experiencing a moderate to severe depressive episode may be more likely than adults to have a manic episode within the next few years.[4] Trials of treatment for child and adolescent depression have found high rates of spontaneous remission (as much as two thirds of people in some inpatient studies).

AIMS To improve mood, social and occupational functioning, and quality of life; to reduce morbidity and mortality; to prevent recurrence of depressive disorder; and to minimise adverse effects of treatment.

OUTCOMES See depressive disorders, p 74. In children and adolescents there are developmentally specific continuous measures such as the Children's Depression Rating Scale and the Children's Depression Inventory. Categorical outcomes are sometimes expressed as people no longer meeting specified criteria for depression on a structured psychiatric interview such as the Kiddie-SADS.

METHODS *Clinical Evidence* search and appraisal May 2001.

QUESTION **What are the effects of treatments?**

OPTION **PRESCRIPTION ANTIDEPRESSANT DRUGS**

Two systematic reviews found no evidence of benefit from tricyclic antidepressants in prepubertal children and no clear benefit in adolescents. We found limited evidence that fluoxetine may be of some benefit for child and adolescent depression. We found no evidence about other serotonin reuptake inhibitor drugs. We found little high quality evidence regarding moclobemide. We found no evidence on the effectiveness of non-reversible monoamine oxidase inhibitors. We found no evidence that venlafaxine or lithium are beneficial, although the power of the RCTs was too low to rule out a clinically important difference.

Benefits: **Tricyclic antidepressants:** We found two systematic reviews (search date 2000[6] and search date 1999[7], 9 RCTs, 357 children and adolescents) that overlapped in their inclusion of seven RCTs.

The first systematic review found no significant reduction in non-response with active drug versus placebo (273 people; OR 0.83, 95% CI 0.48 to 1.42).[6] The second review found similar results (330 people; OR 0.92, 95% CI 0.57 to 1.47).[7] Analyses for children (2 RCTs) and adolescents (5 RCTs) also found no significant benefit of treatment (children RR of failure to recover 0.9, 95% CI 0.7 to 1.2; adolescents RR of failure to recover 0.9, 95% CI 0.7 to 1.3), but found a significant difference using the weighted mean difference in depression checklist scores −2.3, 95% CI −3.3 to −1.4) but not in children.[6] **Pulsed intravenous clomipramine:** See glossary, p 72. We found no systematic review. One small RCT (including 16 non-suicidal adolescent outpatients with major depression) found that significantly more people (7/8) responded to intravenous clomipramine 200 mg than to saline (3/8).[8] **Monoamine oxidase inhibitors:** We found no systematic review. In one small RCT, 20 adolescents treated with moclobemide showed greater improvement on one clinician rated scale than those treated with placebo, but not on other clinician rated and self-reported measures.[9] We found no RCTs of non-reversible monoamine oxidase inhibitors. **Selective serotonin reuptake inhibitors:** We found one systematic review (search date 1998, 2 RCTs, 126 children) addressing both adults and children.[10] The first RCT in the systematic review (40 adolescents, of whom 30 completed the trial) found no benefit on the Clinical Global Impressions scale. The second RCT (96 children and adolescents) found significantly more children and adolescents improved with fluoxetine (27/48) than with placebo (16/48) on the Clinical Global Impressions scale (RR of failure to recover 0.66, 95% CI 0.45 to 0.96), and there was greater mean improvement with active treatment on the self report Children's Depressive Rating Scale (34% v 18%; P < 0.01) but not on other measures. The systematic review did not pool results from the two RCTs. However, combination of the results for clinician global rating, using a fixed effects model, found an insignificant/borderline significant relative risk for non-improvement (0.7, 95% CI 0.49 to 1.00). **Selective noradrenergic reuptake inhibitors:** We found one systematic review (search date 1998, 1 RCT, 33 children).[10] The one small RCT compared a combination of venlafaxine and psychotherapy with a combination of placebo and psychotherapy. It found no significant difference with regard to improvement. **Lithium:** We found no systematic review. One small placebo controlled RCT compared lithium versus placebo in 30 depressed prepubertal children with a family history of bipolar affective disorder.[11] It found no significant difference of global assessment or of depression scores at follow up.

Harms: See harms of antidepressants under depressive disorders, p 871. We found one unpublished systematic review (see comment below). We found single case reports and case series of toxicity and death from tricyclic antidepressants in overdose and therapeutic doses (see harms of antidepressants under depressive disorders, p 84). Of the 17 children randomised to lithium treatment, four were withdrawn because of adverse effects (3 had confusion, 1 had nausea and vomiting).[11]

Depression in children and adolescents

Comment: One systematic review awaiting publication found that tricyclic antidepressants were more commonly associated with vertigo (OR 8.47, 95% CI 1.40 to 51.0), orthostatic hypotension (OR 4.77, 95% CI 1.11 to 20.5), and dry mouth (OR 5.19, 95% CI 1.15 to 23.5) than placebo.[6] It found no significant differences for other adverse effects (tiredness, sleep problems, headache, palpitations, tremor, perspiration, constipation, or problems with micturition). Further research is needed to determine long term effects of intravenous clomipramine.

OPTION   ST JOHN'S WORT (*HYPERICUM PERFORATUM*)

We found no evidence on the effects of St John's Wort *(H perforatum)* in children and adolescents with depression.

Benefits: We found no systematic review and no RCTs in children or adolescents.

Harms: See harms of St John's Wort under depressive disorders, p 874. We found no evidence on adverse effects in children and adolescents.

Comment: None.

OPTION   ELECTROCONVULSIVE THERAPY

We found insufficient evidence about the use of electroconvulsive therapy in children and adolescents with depression.

Benefits: We found no systematic reviews or RCTs.

Harms: We found no evidence on specific harms in children or adolescents (see harms of electroconvulsive therapy under depressive disorders, p 81).

Comment: None.

OPTION   SPECIFIC PSYCHOLOGICAL TREATMENTS

One systematic review has found that cognitive behavioural therapy increases the rate of resolution of the symptoms of depression compared with non-specific supportive therapies for children and adolescents with mild to moderate depression. We found limited evidence from two small RCTs of interpersonal therapy versus clinical monitoring alone or placement on a waiting list. We found insufficient evidence that family therapy or group treatments other than cognitive behavioural therapy are effective treatments for depression in children and adolescents.

Benefits: **Cognitive behavioural therapy:** See glossary, p 72. We found one systematic review (search date 1997, 6 RCTs, 376 people) of cognitive behavioural therapy compared with "inactive" treatment that ranged from waiting list control to supportive psychotherapy.[12] Cognitive behavioural therapy was associated with increased rate of resolution of symptoms of depression (OR 3.2, 95% CI 1.9 to 5.2; NNT 4, 95% CI 3 to 5): a finding consistent with three non-systematic meta-analytic studies.[13–15] **Interpersonal therapy:** See glossary, p 72. We found no systematic review. We found two RCTs, which compared 12 weekly sessions of interpersonal therapy versus clinical monitoring or waiting list control in adolescents with depression. In the first RCT, 18 of 24 adolescents receiving interpersonal therapy recovered versus 11 of 24 adolescents receiving clinical monitoring alone (RR 1.64, 95% CI 1.00 to 2.68; ARR 0.29, 95% CI 0.03 to 0.56).[16] In the second RCT, 17 of 19 adolescents receiving interpersonal therapy recovered versus 12 of 18 adolescents on the waiting list (RR 1.33, 95% CI 0.94 to 1.93; ARR 0.22, 95% CI −0.03 to +0.49).[17] **Systemic behavioural family therapy:** See glossary, p 72. We found no systematic review. One RCT of family therapy versus non-specific supportive therapy did not find a significant difference in remission rates (29% v 34%).[18] **Group administered cognitive behavioural therapy:** We found no systematic review. One RCT group that administered cognitive behavioural therapy for adolescents with depression produced a significantly higher remission rate among those receiving treatment (67%) compared with those on a waiting list (48%).[19] **Group therapeutic support versus group social skills training:** We found no systematic review. One RCT (47 adolescents) comparing group therapeutic support versus group social skills training found no significant difference in remission rates (50% v 40%).[20]

Harms: See harms of specific psychological treatments under depressive disorders, p 82. We found no report of harms specifically for children and adolescents.

Comment: See comment of specific psychological treatments under depressive disorders, p 82. In the first RCT of interpersonal therapy, sessions were augmented by telephone contact.

QUESTION **Which treatments are most effective at improving long term outcome?**

We found no systematic reviews and no RCTs looking at long term outcomes.

Benefits: We found no systematic reviews and no RCTs. We found no RCTs comparing structured psychotherapy with pharmacotherapy in children and adolescents. We found no RCTs comparing combined pharmacotherapy and psychotherapy with either treatment alone. We found no RCTs comparing different psychotherapies.

Harms: See harms of prescription antidepressant drugs, p 69, and depressive disorders, p 78. See also harms of cognitive behavioural therapy in Table 2 under depressive disorders, p 89.

Comment: See depressive disorders, p 74. We found one prospective cohort study in which adolescents with depression, randomised to cognitive behavioural therapy, systemic behavioural family therapy, or non-directive supportive therapy (see glossary, p 72) were assessed at 3 monthly intervals for the first 12 months and then once again at 24 months. The study found no significant difference between the groups. Of 106 adolescents, 38% experienced sustained recovery, 21% experienced persistent depression, and 41% had a relapsing course.[21]

Depression in children and adolescents

GLOSSARY

Cognitive behavioural therapy A brief (20 sessions over 12–16 wks) structured treatment aimed at changing the dysfunctional beliefs and negative automatic thoughts that characterise depressive disorders.[22] Cognitive behavioural therapy requires a high level of training in the therapist, and has been adapted for children and adolescents suffering depression. A course of treatment is characterised by 8–12 weekly sessions, in which the therapist and the child collaborate to solve current difficulties. The treatment is structured and often directed by a manual. Treatment generally includes cognitive elements, such as the challenging of negativistic thoughts, and behavioural elements, such as structuring time to engage in pleasurable activity.

Interpersonal therapy A standardised form of brief psychotherapy (usually 12–16 weekly sessions) intended primarily for outpatients with unipolar non-psychotic depressive disorders. It focuses on improving the individual's interpersonal functioning and identifying the problems associated with the onset of the depressive episode.[23] In children and adolescents, interpersonal therapy has been adapted for adolescents to address common adolescent developmental issues, for example separation from parents, exploration of authority in relationship to parents, development of dyadic interpersonal relationships, initial experience with the death of a relative or friend, and peer pressure.

Non-directive supportive therapy See brief, non-directive counselling under depressive disorders, p 875.

Pulsed intravenous clomipramine An intravenous loading procedure for clomipramine.

Systemic behavioural family therapy A combination of two treatment approaches that have been used effectively for dysfunctional families. In the first phase of treatment, the therapist clarifies the concerns that brought the family into treatment, and provides a series of reframing statements designed to optimise engagement in therapy and identification of dysfunctional behaviour patterns (systemic therapy). In the second phase, the family members focus on communication and problem solving skills and the alteration of family interactional patterns (family behaviour therapy).

REFERENCES

1. Costello EJ, Angold A, Burns BJ, et al. The Great Smoky Mountains Study of Youth. Goals, design, methods, and the prevalence of DSM-III-R disorders. *Arch Gen Psychiatry* 1996;53: 1129–1136.
2. Costello EJ. Developments in child psychiatric epidemiology. *J Am Acad Child Adolesc Psychiatry* 1989;28:836–841.
3. Lewinsohn PM, Rohde P, Seely JR. Major depressive disorder in older adolescents: prevalence, risk factors, and clinical implications. *Clin Psychol Rev* 1998;18:765–794.
4. Birmaher B, Ryan ND, Williamson DE, Brent DA. Childhood and adolescent depression: a review of the past 10 years, Part I. *J Am Acad Child Adolesc Psychiatry* 1996;35:1427–1439.
5. Geller B, Fox LW, Fletcher M. Effect of tricyclic antidepressants on switching to mania and on the onset of bipolarity in depressed 6- to 12-year-olds. *J Am Acad Child Adolesc Psychiatry* 1993; 32:43–50.
6. Hazell P, O'Connell D, Heathcote D, Henry D. Tricyclic drugs for depression in children and adolescents. In: The Cochrane Library, Issue 2, 2001. Oxford: Update Software. Search date 2000; primary sources Medline, Excerpta Medica, and Cochrane trials database.
7. Maneeton N, Srisurapanont M. Tricyclic antidepressants for depressive disorders in children and adolescents: A meta-analysis of randomized-controlled trials. *J Med Assoc Thai* 2000;83:1367–1374. Search date October 1999; primary sources Medline, Controlled Clinical Trials Register, and hand searches of the reference lists of identified papers and a previous meta-analyisis.
8. Sallee FR, Vrindavanam NS, Deas-Nesmith D, Carson SW, Sethuraman G. Pulse intravenous clomipramine for depressed adolescents: double-blind, controlled trial. *Am J Psychiatry* 1997;154: 668–673.
9. Avci A, Diler RS, Kibar M, Sezgin F. Comparison of moclobemide and placebo in young adolescents with major depressive disorder. *Ann Med Sci* 1999;8:31–40.
10. Williams JW, Mulrow CD, Chiquette E, Noel PH, Aguilar C, Cornell J. A systematic review of newer pharmacotherapies for depression in adults: evidence report summary. *Ann Intern Med* 2000; 132:743–756. Search date 1998; primary sources Medline, Embase, Psychlit, Lilacs, Psyindex, Sigle, Cinahl, Biological Abstracts, Cochrane Controlled Trials, hand searches, and personal contacts.
11. Geller B, Cooper TB, Zimerman B, et al. Lithium for prepubertal depressed children with family

Mental health

history predictors of future bipolarity: a double-blind, placebo-controlled study. *J Affect Disord* 1998;51:165–175.

12. Harrington R, Whittaker J, Shoebridge P, Campbell F. Systematic review of efficacy of cognitive behavioural therapies in childhood and adolescent depressive disorder. *BMJ* 1998;316:1559–1563. Search date 1997; primary sources Medline, Psychlit, Cochrane, and hand searches of reference lists, book chapters, conference proceedings, and relevant journals in the field.

13. Lewinsohn PM, Clarke GN. Psychosocial treatments for adolescent depression. *Clin Psychol Rev* 1999;19:329–342.

14. Reinecke MA, Ryan NE, DuBois DL. Cognitive-behavioral therapy of depression and depressive symptoms during adolescence: a review and meta-analysis. *J Am Acad Child Adolesc Psychiatry* 1998;37:26–34.

15. Mendez Carrillo FX, Moreno PJ, Sanchez-Meca J, Olivares J, Espada JP. Effectiveness of psychological treatment for child and adolescent depression: a qualitative review of two decades of research. *Psicol Conductual* 2000;8:487–510.

16. Mufson L, Weissman MM, Moreau D, Garfinkel R. Efficacy of interpersonal psychotherapy for depressed adolescents. *Arch Gen Psychiatry* 1999;56:573–579.

17. Rossello J, Bernal G. The efficacy of cognitive-behavioral and interpersonal treatments for depression in Puerto Rican adolescents. *J Consult Clin Psychol* 1999;67:734–745.

18. Brent DA, Holder D, Kolko D, et al. A clinical psychotherapy trial for adolescent depression comparing cognitive, family, and supportive therapy. *Arch Gen Psychiatry* 1997;54:877–885.

19. Clarke GN, Rohde P, Lewinsohn PM, Hops H, Seeley JR. Cognitive-behavioral treatment of adolescent depression: efficacy of acute group treatment and booster sessions. *J Am Acad Child Adolesc Psychiatry* 1999;38:272–279.

20. Fine S, Forth A, Gilbert M, Haley G. Group therapy for adolescent depressive disorder: a comparison of social skills and therapeutic support. *J Am Acad Child Adolesc Psychiatry* 1991;30:79–85.

21. Birmaher B, Brent DA, Kolko D, et al. Clinical outcome after short-term psychotherapy for adolescents with major depressive disorder. *Arch Gen Psychiatry* 2000;57:29–36.

22. Haaga DAF, Beck AT. Cognitive therapy. In: Paykel ES, ed. *Handbook of affective disorders.* Edinburgh: Churchill Livingstone, 1992;511–523.

23. Klerman GL, Weissman H. Interpersonal psychotherapy. In: Paykel ES, ed. *Handbook of affective disorders.* Edinburgh: Churchill Livingstone, 1992;501–510.

Philip Hazell

Conjoint Professor of Child and Adolescent Psychiatry/Director Child and Youth Mental Health Service
University of Newcastle
New South Wales
Australia

Competing interests: The author has been paid a fee by Pfizer, the manufacturer of sertraline, for speaking to general practitioners about the evidence for the treatment of depression in young people. The author's service has been in receipt of funding from Eli Lilly to participate in a relapse prevention trial of tomoxetine for attention deficit hyperactivity disorder.

Depressive disorders

Search date May 2001

John Geddes and Rob Butler

INTERVENTIONS

Key Messages

- Systematic reviews have found that antidepressant drugs versus placebo are effective in acute treatment of all grades of depressive disorders, in all common treatment settings, and in people with or without co-existent physical illness. We found no evidence of a clinically significant difference in the benefits of different antidepressant drugs, although drugs vary in adverse effects.

- Five RCTs found limited evidence that collaborative working between primary care physicians and psychiatrists, case management, telephone support, or patient education improved the effectiveness of drug treatment.

- One systematic review of mixed quality RCTs has found that St John's Wort is an effective treatment for mild to moderate depression.

- Two systematic reviews have found that electroconvulsive therapy is effective in treating depression.

- One large RCT has found that interpersonal therapy compared with placebo or no treatment improves the symptoms of mild to moderate depression. Less robust RCTs have found that problem solving therapy compared with placebo is also effective.

- One systematic review has found that cognitive therapy compared with placebo reduces the symptoms of depression.

- We found no reliable evidence that one type of treatment (drug or non-drug) is superior to another. Limited evidence found that combining drug and psychological treatments may have significant additional benefits in severe but not in mild to moderate depression.

- We found limited evidence about other treatments, including exercise, bibliotherapy, befriending, and non-directive counselling.

- Of the interventions examined, prescription antidepressant drugs are the only treatment for which there is good evidence of effectiveness in severe and psychotic depressive disorders. We found no RCTs comparing drug and non-drug treatments in severe depressive disorders.

- One systematic review and subsequent RCTs have found that continuing antidepressant drug treatment for 4–6 months after recovery reduces risk of relapse.

- We found no evidence of a difference in long term benefits between treatments.

DEFINITION **Depressive disorders** are characterised by persistent low mood, loss of interest and enjoyment, and reduced energy. They often impair function. **Older adults:** Older adults are generally defined as people aged 65 years or older. The presentation of depression in older adults may be atypical: low mood may be masked and anxiety or memory impairment may be the principal presenting symptoms. Dementia should be considered in the differential diagnosis of depression in older adults.[1]

INCIDENCE/ **Younger adults:** Depressive disorders are common, with a preva-
PREVALENCE lence of major depression between 5% and 10% of people seen in primary care settings.[2] Two to three times as many people may have depressive symptoms but do not meet criteria for major depression. Women are affected twice as often as men. Depressive disorders are the fourth most important cause of disability worldwide and they are expected to become the second most important cause by the year 2020.[3,4] **Older adults:** Between 10% and 15% of older people have significant depressive symptomatology, although major depression is relatively rare in older adults.[5]

AETIOLOGY/ The causes are uncertain but include both childhood events and
RISK FACTORS current psychosocial adversity.

PROGNOSIS About half of people suffering a first episode of major depressive disorder experience further symptoms in the next 10 years.[6] Different levels of severity[7,8] indicate different prognosis and treatment. **Mild to moderate depression** is characterised by depressive symptoms and some functional impairment. Many people recover in the short term but about half experience recurrent symptoms. **Severe depression** is characterised by additional agitation or psychomotor retardation with marked somatic symptoms. In this review, treatments are considered to have been evaluated in severe depression if the RCTs included inpatients. **Psychotic depression** is characterised by additional hallucinations, delusions, or both. **Older adults:** The prognosis may be especially poor in elderly people with a chronic or relapsing course.[9]

AIMS To improve mood, social and occupational functioning, and quality of life; to reduce morbidity and mortality; to prevent recurrence of depressive disorder; and to minimise adverse effects of treatment.

OUTCOMES   Depressive symptoms rated by the depressed person and clinician, social functioning, occupational functioning, quality of life, admission to hospital, rates of self harm, relapse of depressive symptoms, rates of adverse events. Trials often use continuous scales to measure depressive symptoms (such as the Hamilton Depression Rating Scale and the Beck Depression Inventory). Clinician reports and self reported global outcome measures are also used. Changes in continuous measures can be dealt with in two ways. They can be dichotomised in an arbitrary but clinically helpful manner (e.g. taking a reduction in depressive symptoms of more than 50% as an end point), which allows results to be expressed as relative risks and numbers needed to treat. Alternatively, they can be treated as continuous variables, as is done for systematic analysis. In this case, the pooled estimate of effect (the effect size) expresses the degree of overlap between the range of scores in the control and experimental groups. The effect size can be used to estimate the proportion of people in the control group who had a poorer outcome than the average person in the experimental group a proportion of 50% indicates that the treatment has no effect. **Older adults:** The Hamilton Depression Rating Scale is not ideal for older people because it includes a number of somatic items that may be positive in older people who are not depressed. It has been the most widely used scale, although specific scales for elderly people (such as the Geriatric Depression Scale) avoid somatic items.

METHODS   A validated search for systematic reviews and RCTs was conducted between May and September 1998 from the Cochrane Database of Systematic Reviews and the Database of Abstract of Reviews of Effectiveness, *Best Evidence* and *Evidence-Based Mental Health*, Medline, Psychlit, and Embase. Studies were included by using epidemiological criteria and relevance to the clinical question. A *Clinical Evidence* search and appraisal was conducted in May 2001, including a search for data on depression in older adults. To date, few studies have concentrated on older adults as a separate subgroup. Most published evidence for the efficacy of antidepressants includes all ages over 16 years or is limited to people aged under 65 years.

QUESTION   What are the effects of treatments?

OPTION   PRESCRIPTION ANTIDEPRESSANT DRUGS

Younger adults: systematic reviews have found that antidepressant drugs are effective in acute treatment of all grades of depressive disorders. We found no clinically significant difference in effectiveness between different kinds of antidepressant drug. However, the drugs differ in their adverse event profiles. On average, people seem to tolerate selective serotonin reuptake inhibitors (SSRIs) a little more than older drugs, but the difference was small. We found no strong evidence that fluoxetine was associated with increased risk of suicide. Abrupt withdrawal of SSRIs is associated with symptoms, including dizziness and rhinitis, and this is more likely, with drugs with a short half life, such as paroxetine. Older

adults: one systematic review has found that heterocyclic antidepressants and SSRIs are effective in the short term in older people with mild to moderate depression. However, overall treatment effects were modest.

Benefits:
In younger adults; versus placebo: We found two systematic reviews.[10,11] The first review (search date not stated, 49 RCTs in people with depressive disorder) included five RCTs in people admitted to hospital (probably more severely ill); 40 RCTs in a setting outside hospital; one in both settings; and three that did not specify the setting.[10] Each RCT compared two antidepressant drugs and included a placebo control group. The review found a mean effect size of 0.50 for antidepressant drugs versus placebo, which means that 69% of those taking placebo did worse than the average person taking antidepressants. Antidepressants were more effective in those with depressive disorders diagnosed according to standard criteria (mainly *Diagnostic and Statistical Manual of Mental Disorders*, 3rd edition, revised [DSM-III-R]). The second systematic review (search date 1997, 15 RCTs, 1871 people) compared antidepressant versus placebo in people with dysthymia (chronic mild depressive disorder).[11] Response to treatment was about twice as likely in the antidepressant group (RR versus placebo 1.9, 95% CI 1.6 to 2.3; NNT 4, 95% CI 3 to 5). **Tricyclic antidepressants (TCAs) versus SSRIs:** We found three systematic reviews (search dates 1999,[12] 1997,[13] and 1998[14]) comparing SSRIs with TCAs. These found no significant difference in effectiveness overall. SSRIs seem to be slightly more acceptable overall as measured by the number of people who withdrew from clinical trials (RR 0.88, 95% CI 0.83 to 0.93; NNT 26).[12] The third systematic review (search date 1998, 28 RCTs, 5940 people) compared the efficacy in primary care of newer antidepressants versus placebo and versus older antidepressants.[14] The average response rate was 63% for newer agents, 35% for placebo, and 60% for TCAs (RR for SSRIs compared with placebo 1.6, 95% CI 1.2 to 2.1). One subsequent small RCT (152 people) compared adherence on dothiepin with fluoxetine over 12 weeks and found no significant difference between the drugs. However, the study was probably underpowered.[15] **Monoamine oxidase inhibitors (MAOIs) versus TCAs:** We found one systematic review (search date not stated, 55 RCTs comparing MAOIs versus TCAs in several subgroups of people with depression).[16] It found that MAOIs were less effective in people with severe depressive disorders but may be more effective in atypical depressive disorders (depressive disorders with reversed biological features — for example, increased sleep, increased appetite, mood reactivity, and rejection sensitivity). **Older adults:** We found one systematic review (search date 1998, 40 RCTs of pharmacological and psychological treatments of depression in people older than 55 years), in an outpatient or community setting.[17] Of these trials, 26 were of pharmacological treatments and 21 of these were placebo controlled. People were recruited mainly from outpatient clinics. There was significant heterogeneity in the study results (P = 0.03). Nine heterocyclic drug studies had a mean difference in Hamilton Depression Rating scores after treatment of −5.78 (95% CI −8.31 to −3.25). Significant benefits were also found for fluoxetine, trazodone, and

phenelzine. Of the 17 drug versus drug comparisons (mainly involving heterocyclic drugs), none showed significant benefit above the others.[17] **Combination therapy with antidepressants plus benzodiazepines versus antidepressant monotherapy:** We found one systematic review (search date 1999, 9 RCTs, 679 people) comparing combination therapy with antidepressants plus benzodiazepines versus antidepressant monotherapy.[18] Combination therapy was more likely to produce a response by 1 week than monotherapy (RR of > 50% reduction on symptom rating scale 1.64, 95% CI 1.19 to 2.27), although this difference was not apparent at 6 weeks. **In people with depression plus a physical illness versus placebo:** One systematic review (search date 1998, 18 RCTs, 838 people) found that antidepressants were more effective than placebo in people with depression and a physical illness (NNT 4, 95% CI 3 to 7). People allocated to antidepressants were more likely to withdraw from the study than those on placebo (NNH 10, 95% CI 5 to 43).[19]

Harms: **Common adverse events:** One systematic review (search date 1996) compared TCAs versus SSRIs in people with all severities of depression (see table 1, p 88).[20] There may also be differences between SSRIs. One large cohort study of people receiving four different SSRIs (fluvoxamine [983 people], fluoxetine [692 people], sertraline [734 people], and paroxetine [13 741 people]) in UK primary care found that reports of common adverse events (nausea/vomiting, malaise/lassitude, dizziness, and headache/migraine) varied between SSRIs (fluvoxamine 78/1000 participant months; fluoxetine 23/1000 participant months; RR versus fluvoxamine 0.29, 95% CI 0.27 to 0.32; paroxetine 28/1000 participant months; RR 0.35, 95% CI 0.33 to 0.37; sertraline 21/1000 participant months; RR 0.26, 95% CI 0.25 to 0.28).[21] Only 52% of people responded to the questionnaire, although this response rate was similar for all four drugs. A study of spontaneous reports to the UK Committee on Safety of Medicines found no difference in safety profiles between the same four SSRIs.[22] **Suicide:** One systematic review (which included trials completed by December 1989) pooled data from 17 double blind RCTs in people with depressive disorder comparing fluoxetine (1765 people) versus a TCA (731 people) or placebo (569 people).[23] There was no significant difference in the rate of suicidal acts between the groups (fluoxetine 0.3%, placebo 0.2%, TCAs 0.4%), whereas development of suicidal ideation was less frequent in the fluoxetine group (1% fluoxetine v 3% placebo, P = 0.04; and v 4% TCAs, P = 0.001). One historical cohort study followed 172 598 people who had at least one prescription for one of 10 antidepressants during the study period in general practice in the UK. The risk of suicide was higher in people who received fluoxetine (19/10 000 person years, 95% CI 9 to 34) than those receiving dothiepin (RR of suicide v dothiepin 2.1, 95% CI 1.1 to 4.1).[24] In a nested case controlled subanalysis in people with no history of suicidal behaviour or previous antidepressant prescription, the risk remained the same, although the confidence interval broadened to make the result indeterminate (RR 2.1, 95% CI 0.6 to 7.9). Although the apparent association may be because of residual confounding, there remains uncertainty about the possible association between fluoxetine and suicide. However, any absolute increase in risk is unlikely to be large. **Withdrawal effects:** We found one RCT comparing abrupt discontinuation of fluoxetine (96 people) versus continued treatment (299 people) in people who had been taking the drug for 12 weeks. Abrupt discontinuation was associated with increased dizziness (7% v 1%), dysmenorrhoea (3% v 0%), rhinitis (10% v 3%), and somnolence (4% v 0%). However, there was a high drop out rate in this study because of the return of symptoms of depression (39%), so these may be underestimates of the true rate of withdrawal symptoms.[25] Between 1987 and 1995 the rate of spontaneous reports of suspected withdrawal reactions per million defined daily doses to the World Health Organization Collaborating Centre for International Drug Monitoring was higher for paroxetine than for sertraline and fluoxetine.[26] The most common withdrawal effects were dizziness, nausea, paraesthesia, headache, and vertigo. **Older adults:** We found no specific evidence on adverse effects in older adults. **During pregnancy:** One systematic review (search date 1999) of the risks of fetal harm of antidepressants in pregnancy found four small prospective studies published since 1993.[27] No evidence of increased risk was found, although the chances of adverse effects with a low incidence cannot be excluded. Decreased birth weights of infants exposed to fluoxetine in the third trimester were identified in one study and direct drug effects and withdrawal syndromes were identified in some neonates.

Comment: The systematic review of older people[17] was limited by the diversity of populations included, and the brevity of the studies. A systematic review is underway to examine the efficacy of antidepressants in older people, including information on adverse effects.[17] Metabolic and physical changes with age mean that older people may be more prone to adverse effects such as falls. As older people take more medications, they are at more risk of drug interactions. Suicide is a risk in elderly people.

| OPTION | CARE PATHWAYS |

We found limited evidence from RCTs that the effectiveness of drug treatment may be improved by a number of approaches, including collaborative working between primary care clinicians and psychiatrists, case management, intensive patient education, and telephone support.

Benefits: We found no systematic review. We found five RCTs.[28–32] The first RCT (217 people with mild to moderate depressive disorders in primary care in the USA) found that, compared with standard treatment, outcomes were improved by collaborative working between primary care physician and psychiatrist, and by intensive patient education. Clinical outcomes were improved only in the subgroup of people with major depressive disorder (91 people; AR of clinical response of > 50% reduction on symptom checklist 74% v 44% with standard treatment; NNT 4, 95% CI 3 to 10).[28] The second RCT (613 people) in a Health Maintenance Organization (HMO) in Seattle compared usual care, feedback (in which doctors received a detailed report on each person at 8 and 16 weeks after randomisation), or feedback plus care management (in which the care manager assessed people with depression by telephone at 8 and 16 weeks, doctors received a detailed report, and care managers facilitated the follow up). The care management group was more likely than those treated with usual care to have a clinically significant reduction in depressive symptoms 6 months after randomisation (estimated event rates 40% of the control group v 56% of the care management group; OR 2.22, 95% CI 1.31 to 3.75; NNT 7).[29] The third RCT (1356 people) in 46 primary care clinics in US HMOs compared a multifaceted quality improvement programme with usual care (including mailed practice guidelines). People in the intervention group improved on continuous rating scales. Among people initially employed, 90% of the intervention group worked at 12 months compared with 85% of the control group (P = 0.05). For people initially not working, there was no difference in employment rates between intervention and control groups at 12 months (17% v 18%).[30] The fourth study, a cluster randomised RCT in UK primary care, compared the effects of a clinical practice guideline and practice based education with usual care and found that the intervention did not improve either detection or outcome of depression.[31] The fifth RCT (302 people with major depressive disorder or dysthymia) compared usual physician care (117 people), usual care plus nurse telehealth (12–14 telephone support calls during 16 weeks of treatment; 62 people), or usual care plus telehealth plus peer support (123 people).[31] People allocated to nurse telehealth were more likely to respond than those allocated to usual clinician care (AR of > 50% reduction in symptoms at 6 months; 57% v 38% with usual care; NNT 6, 95% CI 4 to 18).

Harms: None reported.

Comment: None.

OPTION   **ST JOHN'S WORT (*HYPERICUM PERFORATUM*)**

One systematic review has found that St John's Wort (*Hypericum perforatum*) is more effective than placebo in mild to moderate depressive disorders and as effective as prescription antidepressant drugs. However, these findings have yet to be repeated in fully representative groups of people using standardised preparations.

Benefits: We found one systematic review (search date 1998, 27 RCTs, 2291 people with mild to moderate depression).[33] Of these RCTs, 17 were placebo controlled (1168 people). Ten RCTs (1123 people) compared hypericum (8 RCTs used single preparations, 2 used combinations of hypericum and valeriana) versus other antidepressant or sedative drugs. Hypericum preparations were associated with significant clinical improvement compared with placebo (RR 2.47, 95% CI 1.69 to 3.61) but were not significantly different compared with standard antidepressants (single preparations RR 1.01, 95% CI 0.87 to 1.16; combinations RR 1.52, 95% CI 0.78 to 2.94).

Harms: We found two systematic reviews (one cited above[33] and one other, search date 1997[34]). The review cited above found that adverse events were poorly reported in the trials. They were reported by 26% of people on hypericum compared with 45% of people on standard antidepressants (RR 0.57, 95% CI 0.47 to 0.69) and 15% on combinations of hypericum and valeriana compared with 27% on amitriptyline or desipramine (RR 0.49, 95% CI 0.23 to 1.04).[33] The second systematic review included RCTs and observational post-marketing surveillance studies of hypericum.[34] The most common adverse effects of hypericum in the included trials were gastro-intestinal symptoms, dizziness/confusion, tiredness/sedation, and dry mouth, although all occurred less frequently than on conventional drugs. Findings from observational studies were consistent with these findings. Photosensitivity is theoretically possible; however, only two cases have been reported. Allergic skin reactions seem uncommon.

Comment: The evidence cited above must be interpreted cautiously because it is unclear how closely people in these trials match people in clinical practice, and the preparations and doses of hypericum and types and doses of standard antidepressants varied. More studies are needed on clearly defined, clinically representative people using standardised preparations. Interactions with other drugs are possible and should be considered.

OPTION   ELECTROCONVULSIVE THERAPY

Two systematic reviews have found that electroconvulsive therapy (ECT) is effective in the acute treatment of depressive illness.

Benefits: We found two systematic reviews. The first (search date not stated, 6 RCTs, 205 people with depressive disorder) compared ECT versus simulated ECT (in which people received everything but electric stimulation).[35] People treated with real ECT were more likely to respond to treatment (pooled OR 3.7, 95% CI 2.1 to 6.5; NNT 3, 95% CI 2 to 5; calculated from data in the article). The more recent systematic review (search date 1998), which included 11 additional RCTs published between 1987 and 1998, also found good evidence for the beneficial effects of ECT, but did not quantify its conclusions.[36]

Harms: We found no adequate systematic review of possible adverse cognitive effects of ECT. However, people often complain of memory impairment after ECT. One of the main difficulties in studying this is that depressive disorders also lead to cognitive impairments that usually improve during the course of treatment. For this reason, most of the small studies in this area find an average improvement in people treated with ECT. This does not rule out the possibility of more subtle, subjective memory impairment secondary to ECT. Adverse memory effects would probably vary according to the dose and electrode location.

Comment: The first review cited above[35] did not include several recent RCTs comparing real versus simulated ECT.[37–41] However, the results of these trials are consistent with the review's findings. A further systematic review is in progress.[42] As ECT may be unacceptable to some people, and because it is a short term treatment, there is consensus that it should normally be reserved for people who cannot tolerate or have not responded to drug treatment, although it may be useful when a rapid response is required.

SPECIFIC PSYCHOLOGICAL TREATMENTS

Younger adults: One systematic review has found that cognitive therapy is effective. Weaker evidence from RCTs suggests that interpersonal psychotherapy, problem solving therapy, and brief, non-directive counselling may be as effective as drug treatment in mild to moderate depression (see glossary, p 85). We found limited evidence on the relative efficacy of drug and non-drug treatment in severe depression. Older adults: One systematic review has found that rational psychological treatments (such as cognitive therapy or cognitive behaviour therapy) are effective for older people with mild to moderate depression. However, improvement in people receiving these treatments was no different than in controls who received similar but non-specific attention. This review was based on a small number of studies, the populations varied (although most were community samples), and many of the studies were short term.

Benefits: **Younger adults:** The evidence comparing psychological treatments versus drug or no treatment is summarised in table 2, p 89.[43–46] **Older adults:** We found one systematic review (search date 1995, 14 small RCTs, < 24 people, age > 55 years in an outpatient or community setting) of pharmacological and psychological treatments.[47] It found four RCTs in older adults that compared psychological treatments versus no treatment. None of the RCTs found a significant difference between treatment and no treatment, measured on the Hamilton Depression Rating Scale. It also found six RCTs comparing different psychological treatments. Five of six comparisons of "rational" treatments (such as cognitive therapy or cognitive behaviour therapy) versus no treatment in older adults found significant benefit with treatment. Combined, the "rational" treatments performed significantly better than no treatment, with a mean difference in the Hamilton Depression Rating Score of –7.25 (95% CI –10.1 to –4.4), but were not significantly different from the "non-specific attention" control. None of the RCTs found significant differences in effectiveness between psychological treatments.

Harms: See table 2, p 88.

Comment: Large RCTs are needed in more representative people in a range of clinical settings, including primary care. Because of varying exclusion criteria, the generaliseability of the studies is questionable (see table 2, p 89). Other factors to be considered when psychological treatments are compared with drug treatment include whether serum concentrations of drugs reach therapeutic concentrations, whether changes in medication are allowed (reflecting standard clinical practice), and whether studies reflect the natural course of depressive disorders.

OPTION   SPECIFIC PSYCHOLOGICAL TREATMENTS PLUS DRUG
TREATMENT

RCTs have found that, in severe depression, the addition of drug treatment to interpersonal or cognitive therapy is more effective than either psychological therapy alone. No such effect was observed in mild to moderate depression.

Benefits: We found no systematic review. A non-systematic meta-analysis of six RCTs (595 people) found no advantage in combining drug and specific psychological treatments in mild to moderate depressive disorders, but that in more severe depressive disorders combining drug and interpersonal therapy or cognitive therapy (see glossary, p 85) was more effective than interpersonal therapy or cognitive therapy alone.[48] One recent RCT (681 adults with chronic depressive disorder) compared nefazodone or cognitive behavioural–analysis psychotherapy alone with combination treatment.[49] At 12 weeks, the combined treatment improved the rate of clinical response (at least 50% reduction on the Hamilton Depression Rating Scale and a score of 15 or less; combined therapy v both single interventions, NNT 5, 95% CI 3 to 6).

Harms: We found no evidence of adverse effects.

Comment: A systematic review is needed to address this question.

OPTION   EXERCISE

We found limited evidence from one systematic review and one subsequent RCT that exercise may improve depression.

Benefits: We found one systematic review (search date not stated) examining exercise in depressive disorders.[50] It found that exercise improved depression and that this continued in follow up measures. However, it was difficult to interpret because it included non-randomised studies and did not clearly describe participants.[50] One subsequent RCT (156 people) compared aerobic exercise, sertraline hydrochloride (an SSRI), and combined treatment for 16 weeks. It found that all groups improved on continuous rating scales, but there was no significant difference in overall improvement between treatments. The proportion of people in remission (those no longer meeting criteria for depression or with a Hamilton Depression Rating Scale < 8) was not significantly different across the treatment groups.[51] A 10 month follow up of this RCT[52] found lower rates of relapse with exercise versus medication (see comment below).

Harms: None reported. Sertraline is known to have an adverse effects profile similar to other SSRIs (see harms of prescription antidepressants, p 78). No specific adverse effects were identified in this trial for exercise.

Comment: In the subsequent RCT, about half of the people in the medication group engaged in exercise during follow up, making it difficult to draw firm conclusions about specific effects of exercise treatment. The clinical importance of the observed difference at 10 months remains unclear.[52]

| OPTION | BIBLIOTHERAPY |

We found limited evidence from one systematic review that bibliotherapy may reduce mild depressive symptoms.

Benefits: We found one systematic review (search date not stated).[53] It identified six small short term RCTs of bibliotherapy (see glossary, p 85) in 273 people recruited by advertisement through the media and probably with only mild depression.[53] The mean effect size of bibliotherapy was 0.82 (95% CI 0.50 to 1.15). This means that 79% of control people had a worse outcome than the average member of the group receiving bibliotherapy.

Harms: None reported.

Comment: Further studies are needed in clinically representative groups.

| OPTION | BEFRIENDING |

Limited evidence from one small RCT found that befriending reduced symptoms of depression.

Benefits: We found one small RCT (86 women with chronic depression in London) of befriending (see glossary, p 85). Initial identification was by postal screening of women registered with, but not attending, primary care.[54] It found that the befriended group were more likely to experience remission of symptoms at 13 months (65% with befriending v 39% with control; P < 0.05; NNT 4, 95% CI 2 to 18).

Harms: None reported.

Comment: Fewer than half of the women screened were interested in befriending as a treatment option.

| QUESTION | What are the effects of continuation treatment with antidepressant drugs? |

One systematic review and subsequent RCTs have found that continuation treatment with antidepressant drugs for 4–6 months after recovery reduces risk of relapse.

Benefits: We found one systematic review (search date not stated, 6 RCTs, 312 people).[55] Continuation of antidepressant medication for 4–6 months after acute treatment reduced the relapse rate by nearly half (RR 0.6, 95% CI 0.4 to 0.7). Several more recent RCTs confirm this reduction in risk of early relapse with continuing antidepressant treatment for 6–12 months after acute treatment. **Older adults:** We found one RCT (69 older people who had recovered sufficiently and consented to enter a 2 year trial of continuation treatment [see glossary, p 85]), which compared dothiepin versus placebo.[56] Dothiepin reduced the risk of relapse by 55% (RR 0.45, 95% CI 0.22 to 0.96).

Harms: Adverse effects seem to be similar to those reported in trials of acute treatment.

Comment: We found no adequate systematic review of maintenance treatment (see glossary, p 86), but several RCTs have found that maintenance treatment reduced the relapse rate compared with placebo in recurrent depressive disorder. However, they all have problems with their methods (e.g. high withdrawal rates).[57] A systematic review of antidepressant treatment duration is in progress.[58]

QUESTION **Which treatments are most effective at improving long term outcome?**

One systematic review found no evidence of a difference between treatments in terms of long term benefits. The systematic review and one additional RCT found limited evidence that cognitive therapy may be an alternative to drug maintenance therapy in preventing relapse.

Benefits: We found one systematic review (search date not stated), which identified eight small RCTs examining long term (at least 1 year) recovery or relapse rates after treatment had stopped.[43] The trials compared cognitive therapy (see glossary, p 85) versus antidepressants in people with mainly mild to moderate depressive disorders.[43] Overall, 30% of people[16] treated with cognitive therapy relapsed compared with 60% of those treated with antidepressants. However, the number of people in these trials was too small for this trend to be significant. We found one small additional RCT (40 people) comparing cognitive therapy with normal clinical management for residual depressive symptoms in people who had responded to antidepressants. It also found that at 2 years, fewer people relapsed with cognitive therapy than with antidepressants.[59]

Harms: See harms of prescription antidepressant drugs, p 78, and see table 2, p 89.

Comment: The review did not present information on the proportion of people who recovered and remained well in the long term. The largest RCT found that only a fifth of people remained well over 18 months' follow up, and that there were no significant differences between interpersonal psychotherapy, cognitive therapy, or drug treatment.[45] It is possible that different people respond to different treatments. Further large scale comparative studies are needed of the long term effectiveness of treatments in people with all severities of depressive disorders.

GLOSSARY

Befriending Consists of a befriender meeting the person to talk and socialise for at least 1 hour per week, acting as a friend.

Bibliotherapy Advising people to read written material such as *Feeling good: the new mood therapy* by David Burns (New York: New American Library, 1980).

Brief, non-directive counselling Helping people to express feelings and clarify thoughts and difficulties; therapists suggest alternative understandings and do not give direct advice but try to encourage people to solve their own problems.

Cognitive therapy Brief (20 sessions over 12–16 wks) structured treatment aimed at changing the dysfunctional beliefs and negative automatic thoughts that characterise depressive disorders. It requires a highly trained therapist.[60]

Continuation treatment Continuation of treatment after successful resolution of a depressive episode to prevent relapse.

Interpersonal psychotherapy Standardised form of brief psychotherapy (usually 12–16 weekly sessions) primarily intended for outpatients with unipolar non-psychotic depressive disorders. It focuses on improving the persons interpersonal functioning and identifying the problems associated with the onset of the depressive episode.[61]

Maintenance treatment Long term treatment of recurrent depressive disorder to prevent the recurrence of further depressive episodes.

Problem solving Consists of three stages: (1) identifying the main problems for the person; (2) generating solutions; and (3) trying out the solutions. Potentially briefer and simpler than cognitive therapy and may be feasible in primary care.[45]

REFERENCES

1. Rosenstein, Leslie D. Differential diagnosis of the major progressive dementias and depression in middle and late adulthood: a summary of the literature of the early 1990s. *Neuropsychol Rev* 1998;8:109–167.

2. Katon W, Schulberg H. Epidemiology of depression in primary care. *Gen Hosp Psychiatry* 1992;14: 237–247.

3. Murray CJ, Lopez AD. Regional patterns of disability-free life expectancy and disability-adjusted life expectancy: global burden of disease study. *Lancet* 1997;349:1347–1352.

4. Murray CJ, Lopez AD. Alternative projections of mortality and disability by cause 1990–2020: global burden of disease study. *Lancet* 1997;349: 1498–1504.

5. Beekman ATF, Copeland JRM, Prince MJ. Review of community prevalence of depression in later life. *Br J Psychiatry* 1999;174:307–311.

6. Judd LL, Akiskal HS, Maser JD, et al. A prospective 12 year study of subsyndromal and syndromal depressive symptoms in unipolar major depressive disorders. *Arch Gen Psychiatry* 1988;55: 694–700.

7. American Psychiatric Association. *Diagnostic and statistical manual of mental disorders*, 4th ed. Washington, DC: American Psychiatric Association, 1994.

8. World Health Organization. *The ICD-10 classification of mental and behavioural disorders*. Geneva: World Health Organization, 1992.

9. Cole MG, Bellavance F, Mansour A. Prognosis of depression in elderly community and primary care populations: a systematic review and meta-analysis. *Am J Psychiatry* 1999;156:1182–1189.

10. Joffe R, Sokolov S, Streiner D. Antidepressant treatment of depression: a meta-analysis. *Can J Psychiatry* 1996;41:613–616. Search date not stated; primary source Medline 1966 to June 1995.

11. Lima MS, Moncrieff J. A comparison of drugs versus placebo for the treatment of dysthymia: a systematic review. In: Cochrane Library, Issue 4, 2000. Oxford: Update Software. Search date 1997; primary sources Biological Abstracts, Medline, Psychlit, Embase, Lilacs, Cochrane library, personal communication, conference abstracts, unpublished trials from the pharmaceutical industry, and book chapters on the treatment of depression.

12. Geddes JR, Freemantle N, Mason J, Eccles MP, Boynton J. SSRIs versus other antidepressants for depressive disorder. In: The Cochrane Library, Issue 4, 2000. Oxford: Update Software. Search date 1999; primary sources Medline, Embase, Cochrane Group Register of Controlled Trials, hand searches of reference lists of all located studies, and contact with manufacturers.

13. Anderson IM. Selective serotonin reuptake inhibitors versus tricyclic antidepressants: a meta-analysis of efficacy and tolerability. *J Affect Disord* 2000;58:19–36. Search date 1997; primary sources Medline, and hand searches of reference lists of meta-analyses and reviews.

14. Mulrow CD, Williams JW, Chiqueete E, et al. Efficacy of newer medications for treating depression in primary care people. *Am Med J* 2000;108:54–64. Search date 1998; primary sources Cochrane Depression Anxiety and Neurosis Group Specialised Register of Clinical Trials, hand searches of trials and 46 pertinent meta-analyses, and consultation with experts.

15. Thompson C, Peveler RC, Stephenson D, et al. Compliance with antidepressant medication in the treatment of major depressive disorder in primary care: a randomized comparison of fluoxetine and a tricyclic antidepressant. *Am J Psychiatry* 2000; 157:338–343.

16. Thase ME, Trivedi MH, Rush AJ. MAOIs in the contemporary treatment of depression. *Neuropsychopharmacology* 1995;12:185–219. Search date not stated; primary sources Medline and Psychological Abstracts.

17. Wilson K, Mottram P, Sivanthan A. Antidepressant versus placebo for the depressed elderly (protocol for a Cochrane Review). In: The Cochrane Library, Issue 4, 2000. Oxford: Update Software. Search date June 1998; primary sources Cochrane Depression, Neurosis and Anxiety Review Group, hand searched journals, and reference lists. Review not to be published until 2001.

18. Furukawa TA, Streiner DL, Young LT. Antidepressant plus benzodiazepine for major depression. In: The Cochrane Library, Issue 2, 2001. Oxford: Update Software. Search date March 1999; primary sources Medline, Embase, International Pharmaceutical Abstracts, Biological Abstracts, LILACS, Psychlit, Cochrane Library, Cochrane Depression, Anxiety and Neurosis Group Trial Register, SciSearch, hand searches of reference lists and personal contacts.

19. Gill D, Hatcher S. Antidepressants for depression in people with physical illness. In: The Cochrane Library, Issue 4, 2000. Oxford: Update Software. Search date 1998; primary sources Medline, Cochrane Library Trials Register, Cochrane Depression and Neurosis Group Trials Register, and hand searches of two journals and reference lists.

20. Trindade E, Menon D. Selective serotonin reuptake inhibitors differ from tricyclic antidepressants in adverse events [abstract]. *Selective serotonin reuptake inhibitors (SSRIs) for major depression. Part I. Evaluation of the clinical literature*. Ottawa: Canadian Coordinating Office for Health Technology Assessment, 1997 August Report 3E. *Evidence-Based Mental Health* 1998;1:50. Search date 1996; primary sources Medline,

Embase, Psychinfo, International Pharmaceutical Abstracts, Pascal, Health Planning and Administration, Mental Health Abstracts, Pharmacoeconomics and Outcomes News, Current Contents databases, scanning bibliographies of retrieved articles, hand searching of journals, and consulting researchers.

21. Mackay FJ, Dunn NR, Wilton LV, et al. A comparison of fluvoxamine, fluoxetine, sertraline and paroxetine examined by observational cohort studies. *Pharmacoepidemiol Drug Safety* 1997;6: 235–246.

22. Price JS, Waller PC, Wood SM, et al. A comparison of the post marketing safety of four selective serotonin reuptake inhibitors including the investigation of symptoms occurring on withdrawal. *Br J Clin Pharmacol* 1996;42: 757–763.

23. Beasley CM Jr, Dornseif BE, Bosomworth JC, et al. Fluoxetine and suicide: a meta-analysis of controlled trials of treatment for depression. *BMJ* 1991;303:685–692. Search date not stated; but included trials that had been completed/analysed by December 1989; primary sources not given in detail but based on clinical report form data from trials and data from the Drug Experience Network Database.

24. Jick SS, Dean AD, Jick H. Antidepressants and suicide. *BMJ* 1995;310:215–218.

25. Zajecka J, Fawcett J, Amsterdam J, et al. Safety of abrupt discontinuation of fluoxetine: a randomised, placebo controlled study. *J Clin Psychopharmacol* 1998;18:193–197.

26. Stahl MM, Lindquist M, Pettersson M, et al. Withdrawal reactions with selective serotonin reuptake inhibitors as reported to the WHO system. *Eur J Clin Pharmacol* 1997;53:163–169.

27. Wisner KL, Gelenberg AJ, Leonard H, et al. Pharmacologic treatment of depression during pregnancy. *JAMA* 1999;282:1264–1269. Search date 1999; primary sources Medline, Healthstar, hand searches of bibliographies of review articles, and discussions with investigators in the field.

28. Katon W, Von Korff M, Lin E, et al. Collaborative management to achieve treatment guidelines: impact on depression in primary care. *JAMA* 1995;273:1026–1031.

29. Simon GE, Vonkorff M, Rutter C, et al. Randomised trial of monitoring, feedback, and management of care by telephone to improve treatment of depression in primary care. *BMJ* 2000;320:550–554.

30. Wells KB, Sherbourne C, Schoenbaum M, et al. Impact of disseminating quality improvement programs for depression in managed primary care: a randomized controlled trial. *JAMA* 2000;283: 212–220.

31. Thompson C, Kinmonth AL, Stevens L, et al. Effects of a clinical-practice guideline and practice-based education on detection and outcome of depression in primary care: Hampshire Depression Project randomised controlled trial. *Lancet* 2000;355:185–191.

32. Hunkeler EM, Meresman JF, Hargreaves WA, et al. Efficacy of nurse telehealth care and peer support in augmenting treatment of depression in primary care. *Arch Fam Med* 2000;9:700–708.

33. Linde K, Mulrow CD. St John's Wort for depression. In: The Cochrane Library, Issue 4, 2000. Oxford: Update Software. Search date 1998; primary sources Medline, Embase, Psychlit, Psychindex, specialised databases: Cochrane Complementary Medicine Field, Cochrane Depression and Neurosis CRG, Phytodok, bibliographies of pertinent articles, manufacturers, and researchers.

34. Ernst E, Rand JI, Barnes J, et al. Adverse effects profile of the herbal antidepressant St John Wort (*Hypericum perforatum L*). *Eur J Clin Pharmacol* 1998;54:589–594. Search date September 1997; primary sources AMED, Cochrane Library 1997 Issue 2, Embase, Medline, handsearched reference lists, contacted WHO Collaborating Centre for International Drug Monitoring, UK Committee on Safety of Medicines and German Bundesinstitut für Arzneimittel und Medizinproducte plus 12 German manufacturers of hypericum products.

35. Janicak PG, Davis JM, Gibbons RD, et al. Efficacy of ECT: a meta-analysis. *Am J Psychiatry* 1985; 142:297–302. Search date not stated; primary source Medline.

36. Wijeratne C, Halliday GS, Lyndon RW. The present status of electroconvulsive therapy: a systematic review. *Med J Austr* 1999;171:250–254. Search date 1998; primary source Medline.

37. Johnstone EC, Deakin JF, Lawler P, et al. The Northwick Park electroconvulsive therapy trial. *Lancet* 1980;1:1317–1320.

38. Brandon S, Cowley P, McDonald C, et al. Electroconvulsive therapy: results in depressive illness from the Leicestershire trial. *BMJ* 1984; 288:22–25.

39. Gregory S, Shawcross CR, Gill D. The Nottingham ECT study. A double-blind comparison of bilateral, unilateral and simulated ECT in depressive illness. *Br J Psychiatry* 1985;146:520–524.

40. Vaughan McCall W, Reboussin DM, Weiner RD, et al. Titrated moderately suprathreshold vs fixed high-dose right unilateral electroconvulsive therapy. *Arch Gen Psychiatry* 2000;57:438–444.

41. Sackeim HA, Prudic J, Devanand DP, et al. A prospective, randomized, double-blind comparison of bilateral and right unilateral electroconvulsive therapy at different stimulus intensities. *Arch Gen Psychiatry* 2000;57:425–434.

42. Scott AIF, Doris AB. Electroconvulsive therapy for depression (protocol). In: The Cochrane Library, Issue 4, 2000. Oxford: Update Software.

43. Gloaguen V, Cottraux J, Cucherat M, et al. A meta-analysis of the effects of cognitive therapy in depressed people 1998. *J Affect Disord* 1998;49: 59–72. Search date not stated; primary sources Medline, Embase, references in books and papers, previous reviews and meta-analyses, abstracts from congress presentations, and preprints sent by authors.

44. Elkin I, Shea MT, Watkins JT, et al. National Institute of Mental Health treatment of depression collaborative research program: general effectiveness of treatments. *Arch Gen Psychiatry* 1989;46:971–982.

45. Mynors-Wallis LM, Gath DH, Lloyd-Thomas, AR, et al. Randomised controlled trial comparing problem solving treatment with amitriptyline and placebo for major depression in primary care. *BMJ* 1995;310:441–445.

46. Churchill R, Dewey M, Gretton V, et al. Should general practitioners refer people with major depression to counsellors? A review of current published evidence. *Br J Gen Pract* 1999;49: 738–743. Search date 1998; primary sources Medline, Embase, Cochrane Library, and hand searches of references lists.

47. McCusker J, Cole M, Keller E, et al. Effectiveness of treatments of depression in older ambulatory people. *Arch Intern Med* 1998;158:705–712. Search date 1995; primary sources Medline, Psychinfo, and hand searches of bibliographies.

48. Thase ME, Greenhouse JB, Frank E, et al. Treatment of major depression with psychotherapy or psychotherapy — pharmacotherapy combinations. *Arch Gen Psychiatry* 1997;54:

1009–1015. Pooled results of six research protocols conducted 1982 to 1992 at the Mental Health Clinical Research Center, University of Pittsburgh School of Medicine.

49. Keller MB, McCullough JP, Klein DN, et al. A comparison of nefazodone, the cognitive behavioral-analysis system of psychotherapy, and their combination for the treatment of chronic depression. *N Engl J Med* 2000;342:1462–1470.

50. North TC, McCullagh P, Tran ZV. Effect of exercise on depression. *Exerc Sport Sci Rev* 1990;18: 379–415. Search date not stated; primary sources dissertation abstracts online, ERIC, Psychinfo, Medline, books, and abstracts from meetings to June 1989.

51. Blumenthal JA, Babyak MA, Moore KA, et al. Effects of exercise training on older people with major depression. *Arch Intern Med* 1999;159: 2349–2356.

52. Babyak M, Blumenthal JA, Herman S, et al. Exercise treatment for major depression: Maintenance of therapeutic benefit at 10 months. *Psychosom Med* 2000;62:633–638.

53. Cuijpers P. Bibliotherapy in unipolar depression: a meta-analysis. *J Behav Ther Exp Psychiatry* 1997; 28:139–147. Search date not stated; primary sources Psychlit, Psychinfo, and Medline.

54. Harris T, Brown GW, Robinson R. Befriending as an intervention for chronic depression among women in an inner city: Randomised controlled trial. *Br J Psychiatry* 1999;174:219–224.

55. Loonen AJ, Peer PG, Zwanikken GJ. Continuation and maintenance therapy with antidepressive agents: meta-analysis of research. *Pharm Week Sci* 1991;13:167–175. Search date not stated; primary sources references of textbooks and review articles, Medline, Embase, and review of reference lists of primary studies.

56. Old age depression interest group. How long should the elderly take antidepressants? A double-blind placebo-controlled study of continuation/ prophylaxis therapy with dothiepin. *Br J Psychiatry* 1993;162:175–182.

57. Keller MB, Kocsis JH, Thase ME, et al. Maintenance phase efficacy of sertraline for chronic depression: a randomized controlled trial. *JAMA* 1998;280:1665–1672.

58. Carney S, Geddes J, Davies D, Furukawa T, Kupfer D, Goodwin G. Antidepressants treatment duration for depressive disorder (protocol). In: The Cochrane Library, Issue 4, 2000. Oxford: Update Software.

59. Fava GA, Rafanelli C, Grandi S, et al. Prevention of recurrent depression with cognitive behavioral therapy: preliminary findings. *Arch Gen Psychiatry* 1998;55:816–820.

60. Haaga DAF, Beck AT. Cognitive therapy. In: Paykel ES, ed. *Handbook of affective disorders.* Edinburgh: Churchill Livingstone,1992:511–523.

61. Klerman GL, Weissman H. Interpersonal psychotherapy. In: Paykel ES, ed. *Handbook of affective disorders.* Edinburgh: Churchill Livingstone,1992:501–510.

John Geddes
Senior Clinical Research
Fellow/Honorary Consultant
Psychiatrist
University of Oxford
Oxford
UK

Rob Butler
Lecturer in Old Age Psychiatry
Imperial College School of Medicine
London
UK

Competing interests: None declared.

TABLE 1	Adverse events (% of people) with selective serotonin reuptake inhibitors versus tricyclic antidepressants (see text, p 78).[21]

Adverse effects	SSRI event rates (%)	TCA event rates (%)
Dry mouth	21	55
Constipation	10	22
Dizziness	13	23
Nausea	22	12
Diarrhoea	13	5
Anxiety	13	7
Agitation	14	8
Insomnia	12	7
Nervousness	15	11
Headache	17	14

SSRI, selective serotonin reuptake inhibitors; TCA, tricyclic antidepressants.

TABLE 2 Effects of specific psychological treatments for depressive disorders (see text pp 82, 85).

Intervention	Evidence	Benefits	Harms	Disadvantages
Cognitive therapy	One SR (48 RCTs of psychological therapies [2765 people] mainly outpatients in secondary care; therefore, probably with mild to moderate depression; people with psychotic or bipolar symptoms were excluded); 20 RCTs compared cognitive therapy with waiting list or placebo and 17 compared it with drug treatment.[43]	79% of people receiving placebo were more symptomatic than the average person receiving cognitive therapy ($P < 0.0001$).[43] Sixty five percent of people taking cognitive therapy were less symptomatic than the average person treated with antidepressant drugs ($P < 0.0001$).[43]	No harms reported.	Requires extensive training. Limited availability. RCTs in primary care suggest limited acceptability to some people.
Interpersonal psychotherapy	No SR. One large RCT (people with mild to moderate depression) compared interpersonal psychotherapy versus either drug treatment, cognitive therapy, or placebo plus clinical management of 16 weeks' duration.[43]	Rates of recovery from depression: interpersonal psychotherapy (43%; NNT 5, 95% CI3 to 19), imipramine (42%; NNT 5, 95% CI 3 to 22),[43] placebo clinical management (21%).[43]	No harms reported.	Requires extensive training. Limited availability.
Problem solving therapy	No SR. Several small RCTs comparing problem solving versus drug treatment in primary care in people with mild depression.[45,48]	No difference between problem solving and drug treatment.	No harms reported.	Requires some training. Limited availability.
Non-directive counselling	One SR (5 RCTs, people with depression) compared counselling with routine GP management in UK primary care.[46] One protocol registered with the Cochrane database.	The SR provided quantitative results. No consistent improvement in main outcomes, although RCTs found greater satisfaction with counselling versus routine care.	No harms reported.	Requires some training. Limited availability.

SR, systematic review.

Search date June 2001

Christopher Gale and Mark Oakley-Browne

INTERVENTIONS

Key Messages

- Two systematic reviews have found that cognitive therapy is more effective than remaining on the waiting list, anxiety management training alone, or non-directive treatment. We found no evidence of adverse effects.

- One systematic review comparing psychological treatments has not established or excluded a clinically important difference in the effects of applied relaxation and cognitive therapy.

- Two systematic reviews have found that, compared with placebo, benzodiazepines improve symptoms of generalised anxiety disorder. They increase the risk of dependence, sedation, industrial accidents, and road traffic accidents. They have been associated with neonatal and infant morbidity when used late in pregnancy or while breast feeding.

- One systematic review has found that buspirone increases physician rated improvement. Limited evidence from RCTs found no significant difference in benefits between buspirone, benzodiazepines, or antidepressants.

- One non-systematic review found no clear evidence of benefit with hydroxyzine.

- One RCT found no significant difference between abecarnil and placebo. One smaller RCT found low dose abecarnil was significantly more effective than placebo.

- RCTs have found that imipramine, trazodone, venlafaxine, opipramol, and paroxetine improve symptoms. One RCT found that paroxetine improved symptoms more than a benzodiazepine. Adverse effects of antidepressants include sedation, confusion, and falls.

- One RCT in people with generalised anxiety disorder found that trifluoperazine reduced anxiety more than placebo, but caused more adverse effects.

- We found that β blockers have not been adequately evaluated in generalised anxiety disorder.

DEFINITION Generalised anxiety disorder (GAD) is defined as excessive worry and tension, on most days, for at least 6 months, together with the following symptoms and signs: increased motor tension (fatigability, trembling, restlessness, muscle tension); autonomic hyperactivity (shortness of breath, rapid heart rate, dry mouth, cold hands, and dizziness) but not panic attacks; and increased vigilance and scanning (feeling keyed up, increased startling, impaired concentration). One non-systematic review of epidemiological and clinical studies found marked reduction of quality of life and psychosocial functioning in people with anxiety disorder (including GAD).[1] It also found that (using the Composite Diagnostic International Instrument) people with GAD have low overall life satisfaction and some impairment in ability to fulfil roles and/or social tasks.[1]

INCIDENCE/ PREVALENCE Assessment of the incidence and prevalence is difficult. There is a high rate of comorbidity with other anxiety and depressive disorders.[2] The reliability of the measures used in epidemiological studies is unsatisfactory.[3] One US study, with explicit diagnostic criteria (DSM-III-R), estimated that 5% of people will develop GAD at some time during their lives.[4] The reliability of measures used in cross sectional studies to diagnose GAD are unsatisfactory.[2] A recent cohort study that followed people with depressive and anxiety disorders over 2 years found the diagnosis was consistently maintained in 49% of those initially diagnosed with GAD.[5] One recent non-systematic review found that the incidence of GAD in men is only half the incidence in women.[6] One non-systematic review of seven studies found reduced prevalence of anxiety disorders in older people.[7]

AETIOLOGY/ RISK FACTORS One community study and a clinical study have found GAD is associated with an increase in the number of minor stressors, independent of demographic factors,[8] but this finding was common in people with other diagnoses in the clinical population.[5] One non-systematic review (5 case control studies) of psychological sequelae to civilian trauma found rates of GAD reported in four of the five studies were increased significantly compared with a control population (rate ratio 3.3, 95% CI 2.0 to 5.5).[9] A systematic review of bullying (or peer victimisation) found that bullying was associated with GAD (effect size 0.21).[10]

PROGNOSIS GAD is a long term condition. It often begins before or during young adulthood and can be a lifelong problem. Spontaneous remission is rare.[4]

AIMS To reduce anxiety; to minimise disruption of day to day functioning; and to improve quality of life, with minimum adverse effects.

OUTCOMES Severity of symptoms and effects on quality of life, as measured by symptom scores, usually the HAM-A, State-Trait Anxiety Inventory, or Clinical Global Impression Symptom Scores. Where numbers needed to treat are given, these represent the number of people requiring treatment within a given time period (usually 6–12 wks) for one additional person to achieve a certain improvement in symptom score. The method for obtaining numbers needed to treat was not standardised across studies. Some used a reduction by, for example, 20 points in the HAM-A as a response, others defined a response as a reduction, for example, by 50% of the premorbid score. We have not attempted to standardise methods, but instead have used the response rates reported in each study to calculate numbers needed to treat. Similarly, we have calculated numbers needed to harm from original trial data.

METHODS   *Clinical Evidence* search and appraisal June 2001. Recent changes in diagnostic classification make it hard to compare older studies with more recent ones. In the earlier classification system (DSM-III-R) the diagnosis was made only in the absence of other psychiatric disorders. In current systems (DSM-IV and ICD-10), GAD can be diagnosed in the presence of any comorbid condition. All drug studies were short term — at most 12 weeks.

QUESTION   What are the effects of treatments?

OPTION   COGNITIVE THERAPY

Two systematic reviews have found that cognitive therapy, using a combination of behavioural interventions such as exposure, relaxation, and cognitive restructuring, improves anxiety and depression more than remaining on a waiting list (no treatment), anxiety management training alone, or non-directive treatment. The review did not exclude a clinically important difference. One small subsequent RCT found cognitive behaviour therapy improved symptoms more than applied relaxation. We found no evidence of adverse effects.

Benefits: We found two systematic reviews.[11,12] The first review (search date 1996, 35 RCTs, 4002 people, 60% women) included medical treatment, cognitive therapy, or both.[11] Thirteen RCTs included 22 cognitive behavioural therapies, which involved (alone or in combination) cognitive restructuring, relaxation training, exposure, and systematic desensitisation. Combined results from these RCTs found a significant improvement in symptoms with active treatment compared with control treatments (effect size for anxiety 0.70, 95% CI 0.57 to 0.83 and for depression 0.77, 95% CI 0.64 to 0.90; dichotomous data not available). Controls included remaining on a waiting list, anxiety management training, relaxation training, and non-directive psychotherapy. One year follow up of an RCT found that cognitive therapy was associated with better outcomes than analytical psychotherapy and anxiety management training.[11,13] The second systematic review (search date 1998, 8 RCTs, 404 people) made indirect comparisons of treatments from different RCTs, and found that more people given individual cognitive therapy maintained recovery after 6 months than those given other treatments (participants maintaining recovery at 6 months: individual cognitive therapy 41%, non-directive treatment 19%, group cognitive therapy 18%, group behaviour therapy 12%, individual behaviour therapy 18%, and analytical psychotherapy 0%; P values not reported).[12] **Versus applied relaxation:** We found one subsequent RCT (36 people) comparing 12 sessions of cognitive therapy versus applied relaxation (see glossary, p 100).[14] It found no significant difference in response rates (response defined as improvement to score 3 or 4 on cognitive global impression score, 10/18 [56%] with cognitive therapy *v* 8/18 [44%] with applied relaxation; ARR 12%; RR 1.25, 95% CI 0.6 to 2.4).[14]

Harms: The RCTs did not report on narms.

Comment: The second review made indirect comparisons of treatments from different RCTs.[12] This loses the benefits of randomisation as the populations compared may not be equivalent.

OPTION   APPLIED RELAXATION

We found no RCTs of applied relaxation versus placebo treatment. One systematic review comparing applied relaxation with cognitive therapy found no significant difference in the proportion of people with clinically important improvement of their anxiety scores over 6 months. One subsequent RCT found cognitive therapy was slightly better than applied relaxation.

Benefits: **Versus placebo or no treatment:** We found no systematic review or RCT. **Versus other psychological treatments:** We found one systematic review (search date 1998, 6 RCTs, 404 people) of psychological treatment in generalised anxiety disorder.[12] The six RCTs all used the State-Trait Anxiety Inventory. There was significant variation in the type of cognitive therapy (group or individual) and in the comparison treatments, including applied relaxation (see glossary, p 100), analytical psychotherapy, behaviour therapy, and non-directive treatment. Only one of the six RCTs included a placebo group, and that RCT did not examine applied relaxation. Two RCTs included individual applied relaxation (38 people) and four included individual cognitive behavioural therapy (87 people). The systematic review compared arms across RCTs and analysed the raw data from individual studies to calculate the proportion of people who experienced a clinically significant change after treatment and maintained that improvement for 6 months. Applied relaxation was more likely than individual cognitive behavioural therapy to improve the anxiety inventory after 6 months (52% with applied relaxation *v* 41% with individual cognitive behavioural therapy).[12] No statistical tests of significance were performed by the systematic review, but even if the figures presented are taken at face value (see comment below) then the difference between the effects of individual applied relaxation and individual cognitive behavioural therapy were not statistically significant (recovery maintained to 6 months: AR 20/38 [52%] with applied relaxation *v* 36/87 [41%] with cognitive therapy; RR 1.1, 95% CI 0.8 to 1.6). We found one subsequent RCT (see cognitive therapy, p 92).

Harms: No evidence of harms was noted.

Comment: The State-Trait Anxiety Inventory covers only a restricted range of symptoms, and it may not satisfactorily reflect treatment outcomes in generalised anxiety disorder. It is very difficult to interpret the results of the systematic review because the comparison involves arms from different RCTs. This removes the benefit of randomisation because the groups being compared may have different character-istics. The figures presented in the systematic review produce estimates of relative effectiveness with wide confidence intervals: a clinically important difference has not been established or excluded.

OPTION	BENZODIAZEPINES

One systematic review has found that, compared with placebo, benzodiazepines reduce symptoms. However, they increase the risk of dependence, sedation, industrial accidents, and road traffic accidents. If used in late pregnancy or while breast feeding, they can cause adverse effects in neonates. One RCT found no significant difference between sustained release alprazolam and bromazepam. One RCT found no evidence of a difference in effectiveness between benzodiazepines and buspirone. One systematic review, which looked at long term treatment, found no good evidence that any short term benefit of benzodiazepines was sustained.

Benefits: **Versus placebo:** We found one systematic review (search date 1996, 24 RCTs, benzodiazepines [19 RCTs], buspirone [9 RCTs], antidepressants [ritanserin and imipramine, 3 RCTs], all in people with generalised anxiety disorder).[11] Pooled analysis for benzodi-azepines found a mean effect size of 0.70 (no 95% CIs available). The review found no significant differences in effect sizes between different benzodiazepines, although there was insufficient power to rule out a clinically important difference. **Versus each other:** One subsequent RCT (121 people) compared sustained release alpra-zolam with bromazepam and found no significant difference in effects (Hamilton Anxiety Scale scores).[15] **Versus buspirone:** See buspirone, p 95. **Versus abecarnil:** See abecarnil, p 97. **Long term treatment:** We found one systematic review (search date 1998, 8 RCTs, any benzodiazepine medication, greater than 2 months' duration).[16] The weak methods of these RCTs prevent firm conclusions being made.[16]

Harms: **Sedation and dependence:** Benzodiazepines have been found to cause impairment in attention, concentration, and short term memory. One RCT found an increased rate of drowsiness (71% with diazepam v 13% with placebo; P = 0.001) and dizziness (29% v 11%; P = 0.001).[11] Sedation can interfere with concomitant psy-chotherapy. Rebound anxiety on withdrawal has been reported in 15–30% of participants.[17] There is a high risk of substance abuse and dependence with benzodiazepines. **Memory:** Thirty one people with agoraphobia/panic disorder from an RCT of 8 weeks' alpra-zolam versus placebo were reviewed after 3.5 years. Five people were still taking benzodiazepines and had significant impairment in memory tasks.[18] There was no difference in memory performance between those who had been in the placebo group and those who had been given alprazolam but were no longer taking the drug. **Road traffic accidents:** We found one systematic review (search date 1997) examining the relation between benzodiazepines and road traffic accidents.[19] In the case control studies, the odds ratio for death or emergency medical treatment in those who had taken benzodiazepines compared with those who had not taken them ranged from 1.45 to 2.4. The odds ratio increased with higher doses and more recent intake. In the police and emergency ward studies, benzodiazepine use was a factor in 1–65% of accidents (usually 5–10%). In two studies in which participants had blood alcohol concentrations under the legal limit, benzodiazepines were found in 43% and 65%. For drivers over 65 years of age, the risk of being involved in reported road traffic accidents was higher if they had taken longer acting and larger quantities of benzodiazepines. These results are from case control studies and are therefore subject to confounding factors. **Pregnancy and breast feeding:** One systematic review (search date 1997) of 23 case series and reports found no association between cleft lip and palate and use of benzodiazepines in the first trimester of pregnancy.[20] However, one non-systematic review found that use of benzodiazepines in late pregnancy is associated with neonatal hypotonia and withdrawal syndrome.[21] Benzodiazepines are secreted in breast milk, and there have been reports of sedation and hypothermia in infants.[22] **Other:** One non-systematic industry funded review of eight RCTs of benzodiazepines versus placebo or buspirone found consistent improvement with benzodiazepines. However, recent use of benzodiazepines limited the effectiveness of buspirone.[22]

Comment: All the benzodiazepine studies were short term (at most 12 wks). There was usually a significant improvement at 6 weeks, but response rates were given at the end of the RCTs.

OPTION BUSPIRONE

RCTs have found that, compared with placebo, buspirone increases the proportion of people who improve clinically in the short term. Limited evidence from RCTs found no significant differences in the benefits of buspirone, benzodiazepines, or antidepressants.

Benefits: **Versus placebo:** We found one systematic review of buspirone (search date 1996, 9 studies), but it did not report on effects as distinct from pharmacotherapy in general.[11] One of the included studies was itself a non-systematic industry funded meta-analysis of eight placebo controlled RCTs of buspirone in 520 people with generalised anxiety disorder (see comment below). It found that, compared with placebo, buspirone increased the proportion of people much or very much improved as rated by their physician (54% with buspirone v 28% with placebo; $P \leq 0.001$). A subsequent double blind RCT (162 people with generalised anxiety disorder) of buspirone versus placebo found similar results (55% with buspirone v 35% with placebo; $P < 0.05$).[23] A non-systematic re-analysis by the manufacturer of pooled data from eight RCTs (735 people) found a differential response to buspirone depending on whether the participant had been exposed to benzodiazepines (no previous exposure to benzodiazepine: response rate 59% with buspirone v 31% with placebo, $P = 0.01$; recent benzodiazepine use: response rate 41% with buspirone v 26% with placebo, $P = 0.065$).[22] It did not report if the difference in response rates was significant. **Versus benzodiazepines:** The systematic review did not directly compare buspirone with benzodiazepines. One large RCT (240 people) compared buspirone versus diazepam versus placebo. It found that 61% of people on diazepam versus 54% on buspirone achieved a 40% or greater reduction in Hamilton Anxiety Scale score (significance and raw data not provided).[11] A non-systematic re-analysis by the manufacturer of pooled data found limited evidence of a differential response to buspirone depending on whether the participant had been exposed to benzodiazepines (no previous exposure to benzodiazepine: response rate 62% with buspirone v 65% with benzodiazepines; recent benzodiazepine use: response rate 46% with buspirone v 73% with benzodiazepines; significance not provided).[22] **Versus antidepressants:** See antidepressants, p 97. **Versus hydroxyzine:** See hydroxyzine, p 96.

Harms: **Sedation and dependence:** The subsequent RCT found that, compared with placebo, buspirone caused significantly more nausea (27/80 [34%] with buspirone v 11/82[13%] with placebo; RR 2.5, 95% CI 1.3 to 4.7; ARR 21%; NNH 5, 95% CI 4 to 14), dizziness (51/80 [64%] with buspirone v 10/82 [12%] with placebo; RR 5.2, 95% CI 2.9 to 9.6; ARR 52%; NNH 2, 95% CI 2 to 3), and somnolence (15/80 [19%] with buspirone v 6/82 [7%] with placebo; RR 2.6, 95% CI 1.0 to 6.3; ARR 12%; NNH 9, 95% CI 5 to 104). We found no reports of dependency on buspirone. The RCT found no significant difference in the number of people reporting any adverse effect with buspirone versus diazepam (49% with buspirone v 63% with diazepam). Diazepam was associated with more fatigue and weakness compared with buspirone but less headache and dizziness. The non-systematic meta-analysis did not report on the comparative adverse effects of buspirone versus benzodiazepines.[22] **Pregnancy and breast feeding:** We found no evidence.

Comment: All RCTs in the industry sponsored meta-analysis were sponsored by pharmaceutical companies and had been included in regulatory submissions for buspirone as an antidepressant. Other search criteria were not given. RCT methods were similar.[11]

OPTION   HYDROXYZINE

We found one non-systematic review, which found limited evidence that hydroxyzine improved Hamilton Anxiety Scale scores versus placebo.

Benefits: **Versus placebo:** We found one non-systematic review (2 RCTs, 354 people).[24] The first RCT (110 people) found a significantly greater improvement in Hamilton Anxiety Scale scores on hydroxyzine 50 mg daily versus placebo. The second RCT (244 people) compared hydroxyzine versus buspirone versus placebo. It found that hydroxyzine (50 mg daily) versus placebo had no significant effect on the number of people with a Hamilton Anxiety Scale reduction of 50% or greater (30/71 [42%] with hydroxyzine v 20/70 [29%] with placebo; RR 1.5, 95% CI 0.93 to 2.23; ARR 14%, 95% CI −2% to +29%; not intention to treat). **Versus buspirone:** The RCT also found no significant difference between hydroxyzine and buspirone on the number of people with a Hamilton Anxiety Scale reduction of 50% or greater (30/71 [42%] with hydroxyzine v 26/72 [36%] with buspirone; RR 1.2, 95% CI 0.78 to 1.8; ARR 5%, 95% CI −11% to +21%).

Harms: The second RCT (244 people) found significantly more somnolence (10% v 0%) and headaches (6% v 1%) in people taking hydroxyzine compared with placebo.[24] Overall adverse effects were reported in 40% of people taking hydroxyzine versus 38% taking buspirone versus 28% taking placebo.

Comment: None.

OPTION ABECARNIL

One RCT found no significant difference between abecarnil and placebo. One smaller RCT found limited evidence that low dose abecarnil was significantly more effective than placebo.

Benefits: We found no systematic review. We found two multicentre RCTs.[25,26] The first RCT (310 people) compared abecarnil (7.5–17.5 mg/day) versus diazepam (15–35 mg/day), and versus placebo.[25] No dichotomous outcomes were reported. At 6 weeks there was no significant difference between placebo and abecarnil in Hamilton Anxiety Scale scores or clinical improvement. The second RCT (129 people) compared 3 weeks of treatment with abecarnil (3–9 mg, 7.5–15 mg, and 15–30 mg) versus placebo. Within each group the dose was escalated from the minimum to the maximum over the length of the trial. It found that abecarnil 3–9 mg was more effective than placebo (outcome 50% reduction in Hamilton Anxiety Scale score; AR 19/31 [61%] with abecarnil v AR 8/26 [30%] with placebo; RR 2.0, 95% CI 1.0 to 3.8; NNT 4, 95% CI 1 to 12), but the higher doses were no more effective than placebo (AR 12/31 [39%] with abecarnil 7.5–15 mg; RR 1.3, 95% CI 0.61 to 2.6; and AR 10/22 [45%] with abecarnil 15–30 mg; RR 1.5, 95% CI 0.71 to 3.1).[26] Results were not intention to treat (12/34 [35%] people withdrew with abecarnil 15–30 mg v 4/35 [11%] with abecarnil 7.5–15 mg v 1/32 [3%] with abecarnil 3–9 mg v 2/28 [7%] with placebo).

Harms: Abecarnil (3–9 mg) was associated with significantly more drowsiness than placebo (31% with abecarnil v 14% with placebo; NNH 4), fatigue (12% with abecarnil v 0% with placebo; NNH 9), and equilibrium loss (6% with abecarnil v 0% with placebo; NNH 20).[26] Higher doses were associated with more adverse effects.

Comment: None.

OPTION ANTIDEPRESSANTS

RCTs have found that imipramine, trazodone, venlafaxine, opipramol, and paroxetine are effective treatments for generalised anxiety disorder. Individual RCTs found that they were more effective than benzodiazepines, with no evidence of a difference in effectiveness compared with buspirone. There is a significant risk of sedation, confusion, and falls with these drugs.

Benefits: **Versus placebo:** We found one systematic review (search date 1996, 3 RCTs),[11] and five subsequent RCTs.[27–31] The review found antidepressants to be significantly associated with a greater response than placebo (pooled effect size 0.57; dichotomous data not available).[11] The review pooled results for trazodone, imipramine, and ritanserin, so limiting the conclusions that may be drawn for trazodone and imipramine alone.[11] The first subsequent RCT (230 people) compared flexible doses of imipramine versus trazodone versus diazepam versus placebo.[27] It found that at the end of 8 weeks of treatment all three medications produced significantly more patient assessed global improvement than placebo, but were not significantly different from each other (AR 73% with imipramine v 67% with trazodone v 66% with diazepam v 39% with placebo). The results were not intention to treat (18/58 [31%] people withdrew with imipramine, 22/61 [36%] with trazodone, 18/56 [32%] with diazepam, and 20/55 [36%] with placebo). The second RCT (318 people) compared opipramol (a tricyclic antidepressant with minimal serotonin reuptake blocking properties) versus placebo and alprazolam over 28 days. It found that opipramol was superior to placebo (outcome Clinical Global Impression score of < 2: AR 63/100 [63%] with opipramol v AR 50/107 [47%] with placebo; RR 1.35, 95% CI 1.05 to 1.69; NNT 7; 95% CI 1 to 26), but not to alprazolam (AR 63/100 [63%] with opipramol v AR 67/105 [64%] with alprazolam; RR 1.01, 95% CI 0.79 to 1.25).[28] We found three RCTs comparing venlafaxine extended release formulations versus placebo.[29–31] The first RCT (365 people) compared 75 mg daily and 150 mg daily versus buspirone 30 mg daily or placebo over 8 weeks. Treatment with both doses of venlafaxine found a significant improvement in adjusted Hamilton Anxiety Scale scores against placebo. Response was defined as a 50% reduction in Hamilton Anxiety Scale and "very much improved" or "much improved" on the Clinical Global Improvement. There was no significant difference in response rate for 75 mg daily versus placebo (43/87 [49%] with 75 mg venlafaxine v 35/98 [36%] with placebo; RR 1.38, 95% CI 0.94 to 2.04) or 150 mg daily versus placebo (44/89 [49%] with 150 mg venlafaxine; RR 1.38, 95% CI 0.94 to 2.04).[29] The second RCT compared three venlafaxine regimens (75 mg daily, 150 mg daily, and 225 mg daily) versus placebo over 8 weeks. It found significant improvements in the Hamilton Anxiety Scale, and on the Hospital Anxiety and Depression scale. All doses were significantly better than placebo and were not significantly different from each other. There was no significant difference in Clinical Global Impression Scale. Clinical response was not reported.[30] The third RCT (261 people) compared venlafaxine 75–225 mg daily versus placebo over a 6 month period. Intention to treat analysis (last observation carried forward, 44/127 [35%] on placebo and 60/124 [48%] on venlafaxine completed) found a significant reduction of 40% on baseline Hamilton Anxiety Scale score in both Hamilton Anxiety Scale and Clinical Global Impression Scale, sustained over the 6 months (42% response with venlafaxine v 21% with placebo). We were unable, because of the nature of the analysis and reporting, to calculate relative risk or number needed to treat with meaningful confidence intervals.[31] **Versus benzodiazepines:** We found one RCT (81 people with generalised anxiety disorder) comparing paroxetine, imipramine, and 2'-chlordesmethyldiazepam for 8 weeks.[32] Paroxetine and imipramine were significantly more effective than

2'-chlordesmethyldiazepam in improving anxiety scores (mean Hamilton Anxiety Scale after 8 wks: 11.1 for paroxetine, 10.8 for imipramine, 12.9 for 2'-chlordesmethyldiazepam; P = 0.05). **Versus buspirone:** We found no systematic review. We found one RCT (365 people) comparing venlafaxine 75 mg and 150 mg daily with buspirone 30 mg daily over 8 weeks, with a small placebo arm. All treatments were significantly better than placebo but there was no significant difference between them (venlafaxine 75 mg v placebo, NNT 8, 95% CI 6 to 9; venlafaxine 150 mg v placebo, NNT 7, 95% CI 6 to 9; buspirone 30 mg v placebo, NNT 11, 95% CI 10 to 12).[29] **Sedating tricyclic antidepressants:** We found no systematic review or RCTs evaluating sedating tricyclic antidepressants in people with generalised anxiety disorder.

Harms: One RCT found sedation, confusion, dry mouth, and constipation with both imipramine and trazodone.[27] RCTs reported nausea, somnolence, dry mouth, sweating, constipation, anorexia, and sexual dysfunction with venlafaxine. Most of the adverse effects (apart from dizziness and sexual dysfunction) decreased over 6 months in those who continued to take the medication, which (over 6 months) was the minority.[31] **Overdose:** In a series of 239 coroner directed necropsies from 1970–1989, tricyclic antidepressants were considered to be a causal factor in 12% of deaths and hypnosedatives (primarily benzodiazepines and excluding barbiturates) in 8% of deaths.[32] **Accidental poisoning:** Tricyclic antidepressants are a major cause of accidental poisoning.[33] A study estimated that there was one death for every 44 children admitted to hospital after ingestion of tricyclic antidepressants.[34] **Hyponatraemia:** One case series reported 736 incidents of hyponatraemia in people taking selective serotonin reuptake inhibitors; 83% of episodes were in hospital inpatients aged over 65 years.[35] It is not possible to establish causation from this type of data. **Nausea:** There have been case reports of nausea in people taking paroxetine.[36] **Falls:** One retrospective cohort study (2428 elderly residents of nursing homes) found an increased risk of falls in new users of antidepressants (adjusted RR for tricyclic antidepressants: 2.0, 95% CI 1.8 to 2.2, 665 people; for SSRIs: 1.8, 95% CI 1.6 to 2.0, 612 people; and for trazodone: 1.2, 95% CI 1.0 to 1.4, 304 people).[37] The increased rate of falls persisted through the first 180 days of treatment and beyond. One case control study (8239 people aged 66 years or older, treated in hospital for hip fracture) found an increased risk of hip fracture in those taking antidepressants (adjusted OR, selective serotonin reuptake inhibitors 2.4, 95% CI 2.0 to 2.7; secondary amine tricyclic antidepressants such as nortriptyline 2.2, 95% CI 1.8 to 2.8; and tertiary amine tricyclic antidepressants such as amitriptyline 1.5, 95% CI 1.3 to 1.7).[38] This study could not control for confounding factors; people taking antidepressants may be at increased risk of hip fracture for other reasons. **In pregnancy:** We found no reports of harmful effects in pregnancy. One case controlled study found no evidence that imipramine or fluoxetine increased the rate of malformations in pregnancy.[39] **Sexual dysfunction:** A survey (1022 people mostly suffering from depression; 610 women, 412 men) of people using antidepressants with previously acceptable sexual function has reported the incidence of sexual dysfunction to be 71% for paroxetine, 67% for venlafaxine, and 63% for flovaxamine.[40]

Comment: None.

Generalised anxiety disorder

OPTION   ANTIPSYCHOTIC DRUGS

One RCT found that 4 weeks' treatment with trifluoperazine lowered anxiety more than placebo but caused more adverse effects.

Benefits: We found no systematic review. We found one RCT (415 people) comparing 4 weeks of trifluoperazine treatment (2–6 mg/day) versus placebo.[41] The RCT found that trifluoperazine versus placebo reduced the score on the total anxiety rating scale of Hamilton Anxiety Scale (difference 14 points; P < 0.001).

Harms: The RCT reported more cases of drowsiness (43% with trifluoperazine v 25% with placebo) and extrapyramidal reactions and movement disorders (17% with trifluoperazine v 8% with placebo) with trifluoperazine versus placebo.[41] A cohort study found that in the longer term, rates of tardive dyskinesia are increased the more often treatment is interrupted.[42]

Comment: None.

OPTION   β BLOCKERS

We found no good evidence of β blockers in people with generalised anxiety disorder.

Benefits: We found no systematic review or good RCTs of β blockers in people with generalised anxiety disorder.

Harms: We found no good evidence in people with generalised anxiety disorder.

Comment: None.

GLOSSARY

Applied relaxation A technique involving imagination of relaxing situations to induce muscular and mental relaxation.

REFERENCES

1. Mendlowicz MV, Stein MB. Quality of life in individuals with anxiety disorders. *Am J Psychiatry* 2000;157:669–682.

2. Judd LL, Kessler RC, Paulus MP, et al. Comorbidity as a fundamental feature of generalised anxiety disorders: results from the national comorbidity study (NCS). *Acta Psychiatr Scand* 1998;98(suppl 393):6–11.

3. Andrews G, Peters L, Guzman AM, Bird K. A comparison of two structured diagnostic interviews: CIDI and SCAN. *Aust N Z J Psychiatry* 1995;29:124–132.

4. Jessker RC, McGonagle KA, Zhao S, et al. Lifetime and 12-month prevalence of DSM-III-R psychiatric disorders in the United States: results from the national comorbidity survey. *Arch Gen Psychiatry* 1992;51:8–19.

5. Seivewright N, Tyrer P, Ferguson B, Murphy S, Johnston T. Longitudinal study of the influence of life events and personality status on diagnostic change in three neurotic disorders. *Depression Anx* 2000;11:105–113.

6. Pigott T. Gender differences in the epidemiology and treatment of anxiety disorders. *J Clin Psychiatry* 1999;60(suppl 18):15–18.

7. Jorm AF. Does old age reduce the risk of anxiety and depression? A review of epidemiological studies across the adult life span. *Psychol Med* 2000;30:11–22.

8. Brantley PJ, Mehan DJ, Ames SC, Jones GN. Minor stressors and generalised anxiety disorders among low income patients attending primary care clinics. *J Nerv Ment Dis* 1999;187:435–440.

9. Brown ES, Fulton MK, Wilkeson A, Petty F. The psychiatric sequelae of civilian trauma. *Comp Psychiatry* 2000;41:19–23.

10. Hawker DSJ, Boulton MJ. Twenty years' research on peer victimisation and psychosocial maladjustment: a meta-analytic review of cross-sectional studies. *J Child Psychol Psychiatr* 2000; 41:441–445.

11. Gould RA, Otto MW, Pollack MH, Yap L. Cognitive behavioural and pharmacological treatment of generalised anxiety disorder: a preliminary meta-analysis. *Behav Res Ther* 1997;28:285–305. Search date 1996; primary sources Psychlit, Medline, examination of reference lists, and unpublished articles presented at national conferences.

12. Fisher PL, Durham RC. Recovery rates in generalized anxiety disorder following psychological therapy: an analysis of clinically significant change in the STAI-T across outcome studies since 1990. *Psychol Med* 1999;29: 1425–1434. Search date;1998: primary sources Medline, Psychlit, and Cochrane Controlled Trials Register.

13. Durham RC, Fisher PL, Trevling LR, Hau CM, Richard K, Stewart JB. One year follow-up of cognitive therapy, analytic psychotherapy and anxiety management training for generalised anxiety disorder: symptom change, medication usage and attitudes to treatment. *Behav Cogn Psychother* 1999;27:19–35.

14. Ost L, Breitholts E. Applied relaxation vs. cognitive therapy in the treatment of generalized anxiety disorder. *Behav Res Ther* 2000;38: 777–790.

15. Figueira ML. Alprazolam SR in the treatment of generalised anxiety: a multicentre controlled study with bromazepam. *Hum Psychother* 1999;14: 171–177.

16. Mahe V, Balogh A. Long-term pharmacological treatment of generalized anxiety disorder. *Int Clin Psychopharmacol* 2000;15:99–105. Search date 1998; primary sources Medline, Biosis, and Embase.

17. Tyrer P. Current problems with the benzodiazepines. In: Wheatly D, ed. *The anxiolytic jungle: where next?* Chichester: J Wiley and Sons,1990:23–60.

18. Kilic C, Curran HV, Noshirvani H, Marks IM, Basoglu MB. Long-term effects of alprazolam on memory: a 3.5 year follow-up of agoraphobia/panic patients. *Psychol Med* 1999;29: 225–231.

19. Thomas RE. Benzodiazepine use and motor vehicle accidents. Systematic review of reported association. *Can Fam Physician* 1998;44: 799–808. Search date 1997; primary source Medline.

20. Dolovich LR, Addis A, Regis Vaillancourt JD, et al. Benzodiazepine use in pregnancy and major malformations of oral cleft: meta-analysis of cohort and case-control studies. *BMJ* 1998; 317:839–843. Search date 1997; primary sources Medline, Embase, Reprotox, and references of included studies and review articles.

21. Bernstein JG. *Handbook of drug therapy in psychiatry*, 3rd ed. St Louis, Missouri: Mosby Year Book, 1995:401.

22. DeMartinis N, Rynn M, Rickels K, Mandos L. Prior benzodiazepine use and buspirone response in the treatment of generalized anxiety disorder. *J Clin Psychiatry* 2000;61:91–94.

23. Sramek JJ, Transman M, Suri A, et al. Efficacy of buspirone in generalized anxiety disorder with coexisting mild depressive symptoms. *J Clin Psychiatry* 1996;57:287–291.

24. Lader M, Anxiolytic effect of hydroxyzine: A double-blind trial versus placebo and buspirone. *Hum Psychopharmacol Clin Exp* 1999;14: S94–102.

25. Rickels K, DeMartinis N, Aufdembrinke B. A double-blind, placebo controlled trial of abecarnil and diazepam in the treatment of patients with generalized anxiety disorder. *J Clin Psychopharmacol* 2000;20:12–18.

26. Ballenger JC, McDonald S, Noyes R, et al. The first double-blind, placebo-controlled trial of a partial benzodiazepine agonist, abecarnil (ZK 112–119) in generalised anxiety disorder. *Adv Biochem Psychopharmacol* 1992;47: 431–447.

27. Rickels K, Downing R, Schweizer E, Hassman H. Antidepressants for the treatment of generalised anxiety disorder: a placebo-controlled comparison of imipramine, trazodone and diazepam. *Arch Gen Psychiatry* 1993;50:884–895.

28. Moller HJ, Volz HP, Reimann IW, Stoll KD. Opipramol for the treatment of generalized anxiety disorder: A placebo-controlled trial including an alprazolam-treated group. *J Clin Psychopharmacol* 2001;21:51–65.

29. Davidson JR, DuPont RL, Hedges D, Haskins JT. Efficacy, safety and tolerability of venlafaxine extended release and buspirone in outpatients with generalised anxiety disorder. *J Clin Psychiatry* 1999;60:528–535.

30. Rickels K, Plooack MH, Sheehan D, Haskins J. Efficacy of extended-release venlafaxine in nondepressed outpatients with generalized anxiety disorder. *Am J Psychiatry* 2000;157: 968–974.

31. Gelenberg A, Lydiard R, Rudolph R, Aguiar L, Haskins J, Salinas E. Efficacy of venlafaxine extended releases capsules in nondepressed outpatients with generalized anxiety disorder: a 6-month randomized controlled trial. *JAMA* 2000; 283:3082–3088.

32. Dukes PD, Robinson GM, Thomson KJ, Robinson BJ. Wellington coroner autopsy cases 1970–89: acute deaths due to drugs, alcohol and poisons. *N Z Med J* 1992;105:25–27. (Published erratum appears in *N Z Med J* 1992; 105:135.)

33. Kerr GW, McGuffie AC, Wilkie S. Tricyclic antidepressant overdose: a review. *Emerg Med J* 2001;18:236–241.

34. Pearn J, Nixon J, Ansford A, Corcoran A. Accidental poisoning in childhood: five year urban population study with 15 year analysis of fatality. *BMJ* 1984;288:44–46.

35. Lui BA, Mitmann N, Knowles SR, Shear NH. Hyponatremia and the syndrome of inappropriate secretion of antidiuretic hormone associated with the use of selective serotonin reuptake inhibitors: a review of spontaneous reports. *Can Med Assoc J* 1995;155:519–527.

36. Rocca P, Fonzo V, Scotta M, Zanalda E, Ravizza L. Paroxetine efficacy in the treatment of generalized anxiety disorder. *Acta Psychiatr Scand* 1997;95: 444–450.

37. Thapa PB, Gideon P, Cost TW, Milam AB, Ray WA. Antidepressants and the risk of falls among nursing home residents. *N Engl J Med* 1998;339: 875–882.

38. Liu B, Anderson G, Mittmann N, To T, Axcell T, Shear N. Use of selective serotonin-reuptake inhibitors of tricyclic antidepressants and risk of hip fractures in elderly people. *Lancet* 1998;351: 1303–1307.

39. Kulin NA, Pastuszak A, Koren G. Are the new SSRIs safe for pregnant women? *Can Fam Physician* 1998;44:2081–2083.

40. Montejo AL, Llorca G, Izquierdo JA, Rico-Villademoros F. Incidence of sexual dysfunction associated with antidepressant agents: A prospective multicentre study of 1022 outpatients. *J Clin Psychiatry* 2000;62(suppl 3):10–21.

41. Mendels J, Krajewski TF, Huffer V, et al. Effective short-term treatment of generalized anxiety with trifluoperazine. *J Clin Psychiatry* 1986;47: 170–174.

42. Van Harten PN, Hoek HW, Matroos GE, Koeter M, Kahn RS. Intermittent neuroleptic treatment and risk of tardive dyskinesia: Curacao extrapyramidal syndromes study III. *Am J Psychiatry* 1998;155: 565–567.

Christopher Gale
Consultant Psychiatrist; Clinical Senior
Lecturer
Faculty of Medicine and Health Sciences
University of Auckland
Auckland
New Zealand

Mark Oakley-Browne
Professor of Rural Psychiatry
University of Monash
Victoria
Australia

Competing interests: CG has been paid by Eli Lilly, the manufacturer of Prozac, to attend symposia. MOB has been reimbursed by Eli Lilly for attending a conference and for running an educational programme.

Search date September 2001.

G Mustafa Soomro

INTERVENTIONS

Key Messages

- Systematic reviews have found that serotonin reuptake inhibitors improve symptoms more than placebo. One double blind placebo study found that most participants relapsed within weeks of stopping treatment. We found limited evidence that, in people who have responded to an initial course of fluoxetine, maintenance of maximum dose fluoxetine for 1 year may reduce relapse rates compared to discontinuation.

- One RCT found limited evidence that sertraline is more effective than clomipramine at reducing symptoms. One systematic review and one RCT have found no significant difference between clomipramine and other serotonin reuptake inhibitors. However, clomipramine has more adverse effects than selective serotonin reuptake inhibitors, particularly cholinergic and cardiac effects.

- One systematic review has found that behavioural therapy improves symptoms compared with relaxation. Two follow up studies found that improvement was maintained for up to 2 years.

- Limited evidence from data pooling within a systematic review and one RCT found that cognitive therapy is as effective as behavioural therapy. However, one additional RCT found limited evidence that group behaviour therapy may be more effective than group cognitive therapy.

- One systematic review found no evidence of a difference between serotonin reuptake inhibitors and behavioural therapy.

- RCTs found limited evidence that behavioural therapy plus fluvoxamine is more effective than behavioural therapy alone.

Obsessive compulsive disorder

DEFINITION Obsessive compulsive disorder involves obsessions or compulsions (or both) that are not caused by drugs or a physical disorder, and which cause significant personal distress or social dysfunction. **Obsessions** are recurrent and persistent ideas, images, or impulses that cause pronounced anxiety and that the person perceives to be self produced. **Compulsions** are intentional repetitive behaviours or mental acts performed in response to obsessions or according to certain rules, and are aimed at reducing distress or preventing certain imagined dreaded events. Obsessions and compulsions are usually recognised as pointless and are resisted by the person. (There are minor differences in the criteria for obsessive compulsive disorder between the third, revised third, and fourth editions of the *Diagnostic and Statistical Manual:* DSM–III, DSM–III–R, and DSM–IV.) [1]

INCIDENCE/ PREVALENCE One national, community based survey of obsessive compulsive disorder in the UK (1993, 10 000 people) found a prevalence of 1% in men and 1.5% in women.[2] A survey in the USA (18 500 people) found a lifetime prevalence of obsessive compulsive disorder of between 1.9 and 3.3% in 1984.[3] An international study found a lifetime prevalence of 3% in Canada, 3.1% in Puerto Rico, 0.3–0.9% in Taiwan, and 2.2% in New Zealand.[2]

AETIOLOGY/ RISK FACTORS Behavioural, cognitive, genetic, and neurobiological factors are implicated in obsessive compulsive disorder.[4–10]

PROGNOSIS One study (144 people followed for a mean of 47 years) found that an episodic (see glossary, p 110) course was more common during the initial years (about 1–9 years), but a chronic (see glossary, p 110) course was more common afterwards.[11] Over time, the study found that 39–48% of people had symptomatic improvement. A 1 year prospective cohort study found 46% of people had an episodic course and 54% had a chronic course.[12]

AIMS To improve symptoms and to reduce impact of illness on social functioning and quality of life.

OUTCOMES Severity of symptoms; adverse effects of treatment; and social functioning. Commonly used instruments for measuring symptoms include the Yale–Brown obsessive compulsive scale and the National Institute of Mental Health's Global Obsessive Compulsive Scale, both of which are observer rated and well validated.[13–16] Most trials use a 25% decrease in Yale–Brown scale scores from baseline as indicative of clinically important improvement, but some studies use a 35% reduction.[16]

METHODS *Clinical Evidence* search and appraisal September 2001.

OPTION SEROTONIN REUPTAKE INHIBITORS

Systematic reviews and three subsequent RCTs have found good evidence of symptom reduction with serotonin reuptake inhibitors versus placebo. One follow up study found that most people relapsed within a few weeks of stopping drug treatment. We found no evidence of different efficacy among serotonin reuptake inhibitors, apart from one RCT that found limited evidence that sertraline is more effective than clomipramine. One systematic review and two subsequent RCTs have found that serotonin reuptake inhibitors are more effective than other types of antidepressants. RCTs have found that clomipramine is associated with more adverse effects than selective serotonin reuptake inhibitors. One RCT found that maintenance of fluoxetine versus replacement by placebo for 1 year did not significantly change the 1 year relapse rate. In people who have not responded to serotonin reuptake inhibitors alone, two small RCTs found that antipsychotics combined with serotonin reuptake inhibitors reduced symptoms.

Benefits: **Serotonin reuptake inhibitors versus placebo:** We found three systematic reviews and three subsequent RCTs. All found overall benefit with serotonin reuptake inhibitors (see glossary, p 111) versus placebo.[17-22] The first review (search date 1994, mean treatment duration 12 wks) compared clomipramine (a non-selective serotonin reuptake inhibitor — see glossary, p 111), fluoxetine, fluvoxamine, and sertraline versus placebo.[17] Two RCTs of clomipramine versus placebo included 73 children, but the review did not analyse these RCTs separately. It found that clomipramine versus placebo significantly reduced symptoms (9 RCTs, 668 people: SMD 1.31, 95% CI 1.15 to 1.47). It also found significantly reduced symptoms versus placebo with fluoxetine (1 RCT, 287 people: change in Yale–Brown scale SMD 0.57, 95% CI 0.33 to 0.81), fluvoxamine (3 RCTs, 395 people: SMD 0.57, 95% CI 0.37 to 0.77) and sertraline (3 RCTs, 270 people: SMD 0.52, 95% CI 0.27 to 0.77).[17] The second review (search date not stated, 8 RCTs including 4 from the first review, 1131 people with obsessive compulsive disorder) found clomipramine was more effective than placebo (SMD 1.31; $P < 0.01$; CI not provided).[18] The third review (search date 1997, 3 studies, 338 people) found paroxetine (a selective serotonin reuptake inhibitor) versus placebo significantly reduced symptoms over 12 weeks (SMD after adjustment for method variables 0.48, 95% CI 0.24 to 0.72).[19] The first subsequent RCT (350 people) compared fluoxetine 20 mg daily (87 people) versus 40 mg daily (89 people) versus 60 mg daily (90 people) versus placebo (84 people).[20] It found significant improvement of symptoms with all doses of fluoxetine versus placebo (improvement of Yale–Brown scale: fluoxetine 20 mg 19.5%; 40 mg 22.1%; 60 mg 26.6%; placebo 3.3%; CI not provided; all P values v placebo < 0.001). Larger doses produced a significantly greater response ($P < 0.001$). The second subsequent RCT (164 people) found that sertraline versus placebo significantly reduced symptoms (mean reduction of Yale–Brown scale 9 points with sertraline v 4 points with placebo;

CI not provided; $P < 0.01$).[21] The third RCT (401 people) compared three doses of citalopram (20 mg, 40 mg, 60 mg) versus placebo over 12 weeks.[22] It found that citalopram versus placebo significantly improved symptoms (AR for > 25% reduction in Yale–Brown scale: 57.4% with citalopram 20 mg v 52% with 40 mg v 65% with 60 mg v 36.6% with placebo; NNT for 20 mg citalopram v placebo 5, 95% CI 3 to 14). There was no significant difference between the three doses of citalopram. **Serotonin reuptake inhibitors versus each other:** We found one systematic review[17] and two subsequent RCTs.[23,24] The review (search date 1994, 85 people, 3 RCTs) found no significant difference in the improvement of obsessive compulsive symptoms between clomipramine and selective serotonin reuptake inhibitors (fluoxetine or fluvoxamine; SMD –0.04, 95% CI –0.43 to +0.35).[17] One subsequent RCT (170 people) found that clomipramine versus sertraline significantly reduced symptoms (8% greater mean reduction in Yale–Brown scale; $P = 0.036$).[23] The second subsequent RCT (133 people) found that clomipramine versus fluvoxamine did not significantly improve symptoms (change in Yale–Brown scale: 50.2% with clomipramine v 45.6% with fluvoxamine; CI and P value not stated).[24] **Serotonin reuptake inhibitors versus other antidepressants:** We found one systematic review[17] and two subsequent RCTs.[25,26] The systematic review (search date 1997, 7 RCTs, 147 people with obsessive compulsive disorder including 67 children/adolescents) found clomipramine versus non-serotonin reuptake inhibitor antidepressants significantly reduced symptoms (SMD 0.65, 95% CI 0.36 to 0.92).[17] One subsequent RCT (54 people) of fluoxetine versus phenelzine versus placebo found the largest symptom reduction over 10 weeks with fluoxetine (mean relative reduction in Yale–Brown scale: 15% fluoxetine, 9% phenelzine, and 1% placebo).[25] The second subsequent RCT (164 people with concurrent obsessive compulsive disorder and major depressive disorder) found that sertraline versus desipramine significantly reduced obsessive compulsive symptoms (> 40% improvement on Yale–Brown scale: 48% with sertraline v 31% with desipramine; $P = 0.01$) and significantly increased the number of people with remission of depressive symptoms (Hamilton Depression Rating Scale < 7: 49% with sertraline v 35% with desipramine; $P = 0.04$).[26] **Serotonin reuptake inhibitors versus behavioural therapy:** We found one systematic review (search date 1997, number of studies and people not stated) that did not make direct comparisons between serotonin reuptake inhibitors and behavioural therapy (see glossary, p 110), but found no significant difference between indirect comparisons of effect sizes of serotonin reuptake inhibitors versus placebo and behavioural therapy versus placebo.[19]

Harms: **Serotonin reuptake inhibitor adverse effects:** One systematic review (search date not stated, 16 RCTs) found a greater incidence of adverse effects with serotonin reuptake inhibitors versus placebo (RRI 54% for clomipramine, 11% for fluoxetine, 19% for fluvoxamine, and 27% for sertraline).[18] An RCT that compared citalopram versus placebo found that nausea, insomnia, fatigue, sweating, dry mouth, and ejaculatory failure were significantly more common with citalopram.[22] Another systematic review (search date 1994) of controlled and uncontrolled studies found the withdrawal rate because of adverse effects to be 11% for clomipramine, 10% for fluoxetine, 13% for fluvoxamine, 9% for sertraline, and 11% for paroxetine.[19] Anticholinergic adverse effects (dry mouth, blurred vision, constipation, and urinary retention), cardiac adverse effects, drowsiness, dizziness, and convulsions (convulsions usually at doses > 250 mg/day) have been reported to be most common with clomipramine,[27–29] whereas selective serotonin reuptake inhibitors were associated with fewer adverse effects but more nausea, diarrhoea, anxiety, agitation, insomnia, and headache.[27] Both clomipramine and selective serotonin reuptake inhibitors were associated with weight change and sexual dysfunction.[27,29] An RCT (164 people) found more people discontinued treatment because of adverse effects with desipramine than with sertraline (26% v 10%; P = 0.009).[26] One non-systematic review of three prospective cohort studies and five surveys found that fluoxetine during pregnancy did not significantly increase the risk of spontaneous abortion or major malformation (figures not provided).[30] The review included one prospective cohort study (174 people) and three surveys, which found similar outcomes with other selective serotonin reuptake inhibitors (sertraline, paroxetine, and fluvoxamine). One prospective cohort study of 55 preschool children exposed to fluoxetine *in utero* found no significant differences from unexposed children in global IQ, language, or behaviour. It included no information on long term harms for the other selective serotonin reuptake inhibitors. The non-systematic review of effects in pregnancy did not make explicit how articles were selected.[30]

Comment: **Additional evidence:** The first systematic review also identified two small RCTs that found no difference in the effects of non-serotonin reuptake inhibitors (imipramine and nortriptyline) versus placebo.[17] One small, observer blinded RCT (30 people) of fluvoxamine versus paroxetine versus citalopram found no significant differences in the effects of these drugs, but was too small to exclude a clinically important effect.[31] **Duration and discontinuation of treatment:** We found insufficient evidence to define the optimum duration of treatment. Most RCTs lasted only 10–12 weeks.[29,32] A prospective, 1 year study found further significant improvement after a 40 week open label extension of the study, with continuing adverse effects.[33] An observational study found that 16/18 (89%) people relapsed within 7 weeks of replacing clomipramine with placebo treatment.[34] However, one RCT (70 people who had responded to a 20 wk course of fluoxetine) found maintenance of fluoxetine versus replacement by placebo for 1 year did not significantly change the 1 year relapse rate or adverse event rate.[35] A subgroup analysis found that the risk of relapse was lower among people taking 60 mg fluoxetine at randomisation compared to people taking 40 mg, 20 mg, or placebo. However, the dose of fluoxetine was not itself randomly allocated, and so this evidence does not establish that the difference in relapse was an effect of high dose fluoxetine. **Effects on people without depression:** The first systematic review found that serotonin reuptake inhibitors reduced symptoms of obsessive compulsive disorder in people without depression (5 RCTs, 594 people; SMD 1.37, 95% CI 1.19 to 1.55).[17] **Factors predicting outcome:** Four RCTs found that people who did not respond to serotonin reuptake inhibitors had younger age of onset, longer duration of the condition, higher frequency of symptoms, co-existing personality disorders, and a greater likelihood of previous hospital admission. Predictors of good response were older age of onset, history of remissions, no previous drug treatment, more severe obsessive compulsive disorder, and either high or low score on the Hamilton Depression Rating Scale.[36–39] Two cohort studies of people with obsessive compulsive disorder found that poor response to serotonin reuptake inhibitors was predicted by concomitant schizotypal personality disorder (see glossary, p 111), by tic disorder (see glossary, p 110), and also by severe obsessive compulsive disorder with cleaning rituals (OR 4.9, 95% CI 1.1 to 21.2).[40,41]

| OPTION | BEHAVIOURAL THERAPY AND COGNITIVE THERAPY |

We found no studies of behavioural treatment versus no treatment. One systematic review has found significant symptom reduction with behavioural therapy versus relaxation, but found only limited evidence of any symptom reduction with behavioural therapy versus cognitive therapy. One RCT found limited evidence of significant symptom reduction with group behaviour therapy versus group cognitive therapy. We found limited evidence of additional symptom reduction with fluvoxamine plus behavioural therapy versus behavioural therapy alone. One RCT found no significant difference between fluvoxamine plus cognitive therapy versus cognitive therapy alone. Two follow up studies found significant improvement maintained for up to 2 years after behavioural treatment, although some people required additional behavioural treatment.

Benefits: **Behavioural therapy versus no treatment:** We found no systematic review or RCT. **Behavioural therapy versus relaxation:** We found one systematic review (search date not stated, 2 RCTs, 121 people) that found that behavioural therapy (see glossary, p 110) versus relaxation significantly reduced symptoms (SMD 1.18, P < 0.01; CI not provided).[18] **Behavioural therapy versus cognitive therapy:** We found one systematic review[18] and one subsequent RCT.[42] The systematic review (search date not stated, 4 RCTs, 92 people) found that behavioural therapy versus cognitive therapy (see glossary, p 110) did not significantly reduce symptoms (SMD –0.19; P > 0.05; CI not available).[18] The subsequent RCT (76 people) found that group behaviour therapy (exposure with response prevention) versus group cognitive behaviour therapy improved symptoms over 12 weeks and the difference had borderline significance (mean final Yale–Brown score: 13.6 with behaviour therapy v 16.3 with cognitive therapy; CI not reported; P = 0.049; 13 people lost to follow up; analysis not by intention to treat).[42] Recovery (defined as ≥ 6 point Yale Brown scale reduction and score ≤ 12) was not significantly increased immediately after treatment (AR 38% with behaviour therapy v 16% with cognitive therapy; P = 0.09), but was significantly improved after 3 months' follow up (AR 45% with behaviour therapy v 13% with cognitive therapy; NNT 3, 95% CI 2 to 9; P = 0.01). **Combination treatment:** We found one systematic review[19] and two subsequent RCTs.[43,44] The systematic review (search date 1997, number of studies and people not stated) did not find direct comparisons between treatments.[19] In indirect comparisons, it found similar reductions in symptoms with behavioural therapy alone versus placebo, serotonin reuptake inhibitors alone versus placebo, and behavioural therapy plus serotonin reuptake inhibitors versus placebo. One subsequent RCT (99 people in an outpatient setting) found no significant differences in symptoms with behavioural therapy versus cognitive therapy versus behavioural therapy plus fluvoxamine versus cognitive therapy plus fluvoxamine (mean change in Yale–Brown scale: 32% with behavioural therapy v 47% with cognitive therapy v 49% with behavioural therapy plus fluvoxamine v 43% with cognitive therapy plus fluvoxamine).[43] Another subsequent RCT (49 people in a hospital setting) found significantly greater improvement in symptoms with behavioural therapy plus fluvoxamine versus behavioural therapy plus pill placebo (number of people with > 35% reduction of Yale–Brown score: 88% v 60%; RR 0.3, 95% CI 0.1 to 0.96; NNT 3).[44]

Harms: We found no evidence from RCTs or cohort studies of adverse effects from behavioural or cognitive therapy. Case reports have described unbearable and unacceptable anxiety in some people receiving behavioural therapy.

Comment: **Factors predicting outcome:** We found two RCTs of behavioural therapy (total 96 people, duration 2.5 months and 32 wks) and two retrospective cohort studies (total 346 people, duration 1 year and 11 wks).[45–48] These found poorer outcome to be predicted by initial severity, depression, longer duration, poorer motivation, and dissatisfaction with the therapeutic relationship. Good outcome was predicted by early adherence to "exposure homework" (that is, tasks to be carried out outside regular therapy sessions involving contact with anxiety provoking situations), employment, living with one's family, no previous treatment, having fear of contamination, overt ritualistic behaviour, and absence of depression.[45–47] Good outcome for women was predicted by having a co-therapist (someone usually related to her, who is enlisted to help with treatment outside regular treatment sessions; OR 19.5, 95% CI 2.7 to 139.3).[48] Two systematic reviews of drug, behavioural, cognitive, and combination treatments for obsessive compulsive disorder are being prepared. **Maintenance of improvement:** A prospective follow up (20 people with obsessive compulsive disorder, specific diagnostic criteria not provided) after a 6 month RCT of behavioural therapy found that 79% maintained improvement in obsessive compulsive symptoms at 2 years' follow up.[49] A prospective non-inception cohort study of behavioural therapy in 21 people with obsessive compulsive disorder (specific diagnostic criteria not provided) found that, after 2 weeks of treatment, 68–79% maintained complete or much improvement in symptoms at 3 months' follow up.[50] In both studies, some people received additional behavioural therapy during follow up.

QUESTION	What are the effects of treatments in adults who have not responded to initial serotonin reuptake inhibitors?

OPTION	COMBINED ANTIPSYCHOTICS AND SEROTONIN REUPTAKE INHIBITORS

In people who have not responded to serotonin reuptake inhibitors alone, two small RCTs found that antipsychotics combined with serotonin reuptake inhibitors reduced symptoms.

Benefits: We found no systematic review, but found two small RCTs that assessed combined antipsychotics and serotonin reuptake inhibitors in people who did not respond to serotonin treatment alone.[51,52] The first RCT (34 people with obsessive compulsive disorder who had not responded to 8 wks treatment with fluvoxamine) compared fluvoxamine plus haloperidol (maximum dose of haloperidol 10 mg daily) versus fluvoxamine plus placebo.[51] It found that those in the combined haloperidol plus fluvoxamine arm were significantly more likely to have met two out of three different response criteria (11/17 [65%] with combined haloperidol plus fluvoxamine v 0/17 [0%] with fluvoxamine plus placebo; NNT 2, 95% CI 2 to 3; P < 0.0002). The second RCT (36 people with obsessive compulsive disorder who did not respond to 12 wks of serotonin reuptake inhibitor) found that 6 weeks of risperidone versus placebo added to the prior serotonin reuptake inhibitor significantly reduced symptoms of obsessive compulsive disorder (reduction in the Yale–Brown scale: 36% v 9%; P = 0.001), depression (reduction in the Hamilton Depression Rating Scale: 35% v 20%; P = 0.002), and anxiety (reduction in the Hamilton Anxiety Rating Scale 31% v 12%; P = 0.007).[52] People in the combined risperidone arm were more likely to have met two of the response criteria (8/18 [44%] with risperidone plus serotonin reuptake inhibitor v 0/15 [0%] with placebo plus serotonin reuptake inhibitor; NNT 2, 95% CI 2 to 3; P < 0.005).

Harms: One RCT of serotonin reuptake inhibitors with risperidone found that adverse effects (sedation, restlessness, increased appetite, dry mouth, or tinnitus) were experienced by at least 10% of people.[52] Risperidone is commonly associated with hypotension and prolactinaemia. Extrapyramidal adverse effects are more common with haloperidol, which can also cause prolactinaemia.

Comment: None.

GLOSSARY

Behavioural therapy Consists of exposure to the anxiety provoking stimuli and prevention of ritual performance.

Chronic Continuous course without periods of remission since first onset.

Cognitive therapy Aims to correct distorted thoughts (such as exaggerated sense of harm and personal responsibility) by Socratic questioning, logical reasoning, and hypothesis testing.

Episodic Episodic course with periods of remission since first onset.

Non-selective serotonin reuptake inhibitor Clomipramine (also classed as a tricyclic antidepressant).

Schizotypal personality disorder Characterised by discomfort in close relationships, cognitive and perceptual distortions, and eccentric behaviour.

Selective serotonin reuptake inhibitors Fluoxetine, fluvoxamine, sertraline, paroxetine, and citalopram.

Tic disorder Characterised by motor tics, vocal tics, or both.

REFERENCES

1. American Psychiatric Association. *Diagnostic and statistical manual of mental disorders*, 4th ed. Washington, DC: American Psychiatric Association, 1994.

2. Bebbington PE. Epidemiology of obsessive–compulsive disorder. *Br J Psychiatry* 1998;35(suppl):2–6.

3. Karno M, Golding JM, Sorenson SB, Burnam MA. The epidemiology of obsessive–compulsive disorder in five US communities. *Arch Gen Psychiatry* 1988;45:1094–1099.

4. Baer L, Minichiello WE. Behavior therapy for obsessive–compulsive disorder. In: Jenike MA, Baer L, Minichiello WE, eds. *Obsessive–compulsive disorders*. St Louis: Mosby, 1998.

5. Steketee GS, Frost RO, Rheaume J, Wilhelm S. Cognitive theory and treatment of obsessive–compulsive disorder. In: Jenike MA, Baer L, Minichiello WE, eds. *Obsessive–compulsive disorders*. St Louis: Mosby, 1998.

6. Alsobrook JP, Pauls DL. The genetics of obsessive–compulsive disorder. In: Jenike MA, Baer L, Minichiello WE, eds. *Obsessive–compulsive disorders*. St Louis: Mosby, 1998.

7. Rauch SL, Whalen PJ, Dougherty D, Jenike MA. Neurobiologic models of obsessive compulsive disorder. In: Jenike MA, Baer L, Minichiello WE, eds. *Obsessive–compulsive disorders*. St Louis: Mosby, 1998.

8. Delgado PL, Moreno FA. Different roles for serotonin in anti-obsessional drug action and the pathophysiology of obsessive–compulsive disorder. *Br J Psychiatry* 1998;35(suppl):21–25.

9. Saxena S, Brody AL, Schwartz JM, Baxter LR. Neuroimaging and frontal–subcortical circuitry in obsessive–compulsive disorder. *Br J Psychiatry* 1998;35(suppl):26–37.

10. Rauch SL, Baxter LR Jr. Neuroimaging in obsessive–compulsive disorder and related disorders. In: Jenike MA, Baer L, Minichiello WE, eds. *Obsessive–compulsive disorders*. St Louis: Mosby, 1998.

11. Skoog G, Skoog I. A 40-year follow up of patients with obsessive–compulsive disorder. *Arch Gen Psychiatry* 1999;56:121–127.

12. Ravizza L, Maina G, Bogetto F. Episodic and chronic obsessive–compulsive disorder. *Depress Anxiety* 1997;6:154–158.

13. Goodman WK, Price LH, Rasmussen SA, et al. The Yale–Brown obsessive compulsive scale. I. Development, use, and reliability. *Arch Gen Psychiatry* 1989;46:1006–1011.

14. Insel TR, Murphy DL, Cohen RM, Alterman I, Kilts C, Linnoila M. Obsessive–compulsive disorder. A double-blind trial of clomipramine and clorgyline. *Arch Gen Psychiatry* 1983;40:605–612.

15. Goodman WK, Price LH, Rasmussen SA, et al. The Yale–Brown obsessive compulsive scale. II. Validity. *Arch Gen Psychiatry* 1989;46:1012–1016.

16. Goodman WK, Price LH. Rating scales for obsessive–compulsive disorder. In: Jenike MA, Baer L, Minichiello WE, eds. *Obsessive–compulsive disorders*. St Louis: Mosby, 1998.

17. Piccinelli M, Pini S, Bellantuono C, Wilkinson G. Efficacy of drug treatment in obsessive–compulsive disorder. A meta-analytic review. *Br J Psychiatry* 1995;166:424–443. Search dates 1994; primary sources Medline and Excerpta Medica-Psychiatry.

18. Abramowitz JS. Effectiveness of psychological and pharmacological treatments for obsessive–compulsive disorder: a quantitative review. *J Consult Clin Psychol* 1997;65:44–52. Search date not stated; primary sources Medline and PsycLIT.

19. Kobak KA, Greist JH, Jefferson JW, Katzelnick DJ, Henk HJ. Behavioral versus pharmacological treatments of obsessive compulsive disorder: a meta-analysis. *Psychopharmacology (Berl)* 1998; 136:205–216. Search date 1997; primary sources Medline, PsycINFO, Dissertations, and Abstracts International databases.

20. Tollefson GD, Rampey AH, Potvin JH, et al. A multicenter investigation of fixed-dose fluoxetine in the treatment of obsessive–compulsive disorder. *Arch Gen Psychiatry* 1994;51:559–567.

21. Kronig MH, Apter J, Asnis G, et al. Placebo controlled multicentre study of sertraline treatment for obsessive–compulsive disorder. *J Clin Psychopharmacol* 1999;19:172–176.

22. Montgomery SA, Kasper S, Stein DJ, Bang HK, Lemming OM. Citalopram 20 mg, 40 mg and 60 mg are all effective and well tolerated compared with placebo in obsessive-compulsive disorder. *Int Clin Psychopharmacol* 2001;16:75–86.

23. Bisserbe JC, Lane RM, Flament MF. A double blind comparison of sertraline and clomipramine in outpatients with obsessive–compulsive disorder. *Eur Psychiatry* 1997;12:82–93.

24. Mundo E, Maina G, Uslenghi C. Multicentre, double-blind, comparison of fluvoxamine and clomipramine in the treatment of obsessive–compulsive disorder. *Int Clin Psychopharmacol* 2000;15:69–76.

25. Jenike MA, Baer L, Minichiello WE, Rauch SL, Buttolph ML. Placebo-controlled trial of fluoxetine and phenelzine for obsessive–compulsive disorder. *Am J Psychiatry* 1997;154:1261–1264.

26. Hoehn-Saric R, Ninan P, Black DW, et al. Multicenter double-blind comparison of sertraline and desipramine for concurrent obsessive–compulsive and major depressive disorders. *Arch Gen Psychiatry* 2000;57:76–82.

27. British National Formulary. London: British Medical Association and Royal Pharmaceutical Society of Great Britain, 1999.

28. Trindade E, Menon D. Selective serotonin reuptake inhibitors differ from tricyclic antidepressants in adverse events (Abstract). Selective serotonin reuptake inhibitors for major depression. Part 1. Evaluation of clinical literature. Ottawa: Canadian Coordinating Office for Health Technology Assessment, August 1997 Report 3E. *Evid Based Ment Health* 1998;1:50.

29. Jenike MA. Drug treatment of obsessive–compulsive disorders. In: Jenike MA, Baer L, Minichiello WE, eds. *Obsessive–compulsive disorders*. St Louis: Mosby, 1998:469–532.

30. Goldstein DJ, Sundell K. A review of safety of selective serotonin reuptake inhibitors during pregnancy. *Hum Psychopharmacol Clin Exp* 1999; 14:319–324.

Obsessive compulsive disorder

31. Mundo E, Bianchi L, Bellodi L. Efficacy of fluvoxamine, paroxetine, and citalopram in the treatment of obsessive–compulsive disorder: a single-blind study. *J Clin Psychopharmacol* 1997; 17:267–271.

32. Rauch SL, Jenike MA. Pharmacological treatment of obsessive compulsive disorder. In: Nathan PE, Gorman JM, eds. *Treatments that work.* New York: Oxford University Press, 1998:359–376.

33. Rasmussen S, Hackett E, DuBoff E, et al. A 2-year study of sertraline in the treatment of obsessive–compulsive disorder. *Int Clin Psychopharmacol* 1997;12:309–316.

34. Pato MT, Zohar-Kadouch R, Zohar J, Murphy DL. Return of symptoms after discontinuation of clomipramine in patients with obsessive–compulsive disorder. *Am J Psychiatry* 1988;145:1521–1525.

35. Romano S, Goodman W, Tamura R, Gonzales J. Long-term treatment of obsessive-compulsive disorder after an acute response: a comparison of fluoxetine versus placebo. *J Clin Psychopharmacol* 2001;21:46–52.

36. Ravizza L, Barzega G, Bellino S, Bogetto F, Maina G. Predictors of drug treatment response in obsessive–compulsive disorder. *J Clin Psychiatry* 1995;56:368–373.

37. Cavedini P, Erzegovesi S, Ronchi P, Bellodi L. Predictive value of obsessive–compulsive personality disorder in antiobsessional pharmacological treatment. *Eur Neuropsychopharmacol* 1997;7:45–49.

38. Ackerman DL, Greenland S, Bystritsky A. Clinical characteristics of response to fluoxetine treatment of obsessive–compulsive disorder. *J Clin Psychopharmacol* 1998;18:185–192.

39. Ackerman DL, Greenland S, Bystritsky A, Morgenstern H, Katz RJ. Predictors of treatment response in obsessive–compulsive disorder: multivariate analyses from a multicenter trial of clomipramine. *J Clin Psychopharmacol* 1994;14: 247–254.

40. Mundo E, Erzegovesi S, Bellodi L. Follow up of obsessive–compulsive patients treated with proserotonergic agents (letter). *J Clin Psychopharmacol* 1995;15:288–289.

41. Alarcon RD, Libb JW, Spitler D. A predictive study of obsessive–compulsive disorder response to clomipramine. *J Clin Psychopharmacol* 1993;13: 210–213.

42. McLean PD, Whittal ML, Thordarson DS, et al. Cognitive versus behavior therapy in the group treatment of obsessive-compulsive disorder. *J Consult Clin Psychol* 2001;69:205–214.

43. van Balkom AJ, de Haan E, van Oppen P, et al. Cognitive and behavioral therapies alone versus in combination with fluvoxamine in the treatment of obsessive–compulsive disorder. *J Nerv Ment Dis* 1998;186:492–499.

44. Hohagen F, Winkelmann G, Rasche-Ruchle H, et al. Combination of behaviour therapy with fluvoxamine in comparison with behaviour therapy and placebo. Results of a multicentre study. *Br J Psychiatry* 1998;35(suppl):71–78.

45. Keijsers GP, Hoogduin CA, Schaap CP. Predictors of treatment outcome in the behavioural treatment of obsessive–compulsive disorder. *Br J Psychiatry* 1994;165:781–786.

46. De Araujo LA, Ito LM, Marks IM. Early compliance and other factors predicting outcome of exposure for obsessive–compulsive disorder. *Br J Psychiatry* 1996;169:747–752.

47. Buchanan AW, Meng KS, Marks IM. What predicts improvement and compliance during the behavioral treatment of obsessive compulsive disorder? *Anxiety* 1996;2:22–27.

48. Castle DJ, Deale A, Marks IM, et al. Obsessive–compulsive disorder: prediction of outcome from behavioural psychotherapy. *Acta Psychiatr Scand* 1994;89:393–398.

49. Marks IM, Hodgson R, Rachman S. Treatment of chronic obsessive–compulsive neurosis by in-vivo exposure. A two-year follow up and issues in treatment. *Br J Psychiatry* 1975;127:349–364.

50. Foa EB, Goldstein A. Continuous exposure and complete response prevention in obsessive–compulsive neurosis. *Behav Ther* 1978; 9:821–829.

51. McDougle CJ, Goodman WK, Leckman JF, et al. Haloperidol addition in fluvoxamine-refractory obsessive–compulsive disorder. A double-blind, placebo-controlled study in patients with and without tics. *Arch Gen Psychiatry* 1994;51(4): 302–308.

52. McDougle CJ, Epperson CN, Pelton GH, Wasylink S, Price LH. A double-blind, placebo-controlled study of risperidone addition in serotonin reuptake inhibitor-refractory obsessive-compulsive disorder. *Arch Gen Psychiatry* 2000;57:794–801.

G Mustafa Soomro
Honorary Research Fellow
Section of Community Psychiatry
St George's Hospital Medical School
London
UK

Competing interests: None declared.

Search date September 2001

Shailesh Kumar and Mark Oakley-Browne

INTERVENTIONS

Key Messages

- One systematic review and subsequent RCTs have found that imipramine versus placebo improves symptoms in people with panic disorder. One RCT found that imipramine reduced relapse rates in people with panic disorder.

- One systematic review and one subsequent RCT have found that selective serotonin reuptake inhibitors versus placebo improve symptoms in panic disorder.

- We found no evidence on the long term effects of monoamine oxidase inhibitors in panic disorder.

- Two RCTs found insufficient evidence on the effects of buspirone in people with panic disorder.

- One systematic review and one additional RCT have found that alprazolam versus placebo reduces the number of panic attacks and improves symptoms in people with panic disorder. However, benzodiazepines are associated with a wide range of adverse effects both during their use and after treatment has been withdrawn.

DEFINITION A panic attack is a period in which there is sudden onset of intense apprehension, fearfulness, or terror often associated with feelings of impending doom. Panic disorder occurs when there are recurrent, unpredictable attacks followed by at least 1 month of persistent concern about having another panic attack, worry about the possible implications or consequences of the panic attacks, or a significant behavioural change related to the attacks.[1] The term panic disorder excludes panic attacks attributable to the direct physiological effects of a general medical condition, substance, or another mental disorder. Panic disorder is sometimes categorised as with or without agoraphobia.[1] Alternative categorisations focus on phobic anxiety disorders and specify agoraphobia with or without panic disorder.[2]

INCIDENCE/ Panic disorder often starts around 20 years of age (between late
PREVALENCE adolescence and the mid 30s).[3] Lifetime prevalence is between 1–3%, and panic disorder is more common in women than in men.[4] An Australian community study found 1 month prevalence rates for panic disorder (with or without agoraphobia) of 0.4% using ICD-10 diagnostic criteria and of 0.5% using DSM-IV diagnostic criteria.[5]

AETIOLOGY/ Stressful life events tend to precede the onset of panic disorder,[6,7]
RISK FACTORS although a negative interpretation of these events in addition to their occurrence has been suggested as an important aetiological factor.[8] Panic disorder is associated with major depression,[9] social phobia, generalised anxiety disorder, obsessive compulsive disorder,[10] and a substantial risk of drug and alcohol abuse.[11] It is also associated with avoidant, histrionic, and dependent personality disorders.[10]

PROGNOSIS The severity of symptoms in people with panic disorder fluctuates considerably, with periods of no attacks, or only mild attacks with few symptoms, being common. There is often a long delay between the initial onset of symptoms and presentation for treatment. Recurrent attacks may continue for a number of years, especially if associated with agoraphobia. Reduced social or occupational functioning varies among people with panic disorder and is worse in people with associated agoraphobia. Panic disorder is also associated with an increased rate of attempted but unsuccessful suicide.[12]

AIMS To reduce the severity and frequency of panic attacks, phobic avoidance, and anticipatory anxiety; to improve social and occupational functioning, with minimal adverse effects of treatment.

OUTCOMES Measures of panic attacks, agoraphobia, and associated disability (self reported and clinician rated, before and after treatment, and longer term) using general scales or specific scales for panic disorder (e.g. the panic and agoraphobia scale, the mobility inventory for agoraphobia).

METHODS   *Clinical Evidence* search and appraisal September 2001. Studies with follow up periods of less than 6 months were excluded.

> **QUESTION**   **What are the effects of drug treatments for panic disorder?**

> **OPTION**   **TRICYCLIC ANTIDEPRESSANTS**

One systematic review and subsequent RCTs have found that imipramine versus placebo improves symptoms in people with panic disorder. One RCT found that imipramine reduced relapse rates in people with panic disorder.

Benefits: We found one systematic review,[13] one additional RCT,[14] and two subsequent RCTs.[15,16] The systematic review (search date not stated, 27 RCTs, 2348 people) compared imipramine, selective serotonin reuptake inhibitors (paroxetine, fluvoxamine, zimelidine, and clomiprimine; see comment below) and alprazolam versus placebo and versus each other (see benefits of selective serotonin reuptake inhibitors, p 116, and benzodiazepines, p 117).[13] It found that imipramine versus placebo significantly increased the number of people judged to have improved ($P < 0.0001$; see comment below). The additional RCT (181 people with panic disorder with or without agoraphobia) compared three treatments: oral imipramine (maximum dose 225 mg; see comment below); oral alprazolam (maximum dose 10 mg; see comment below); and placebo (see benefits of benzodiazepines, p 117).[14] It found that imipramine versus placebo reduced the number of panic attacks after 8 months (results presented graphically, significance not calculated). The first subsequent RCT (56 adults with panic disorder and agoraphobia in stable remission after 24 weeks' treatment with oral imipramine) comparing oral imipramine (2.25 mg/kg daily) versus placebo found that significantly fewer people taking imipramine relapsed after 12 months (see comment below; 1/29 [3%] with imipramine v 10/27 [37%] with placebo; RR 0.09, 95% CI 0.01 to 0.68; NNT 5, 95% CI 3 to 14).[16] The second subsequent RCT (312 people) compared five groups: oral imipramine (maximum dose 300 mg/day; see comment below); cognitive behavioural therapy (see glossary, p 118); placebo; cognitive behavioural therapy plus oral imipramine (maximum dose 300 mg/day; see comment below); and cognitive behavioural therapy plus placebo.[15] It found that imipramine versus placebo significantly increased the number of people judged to have responded using the panic disorder severity scale after 6 months (38% response rate with imipramine v 13% response rate with placebo; absolute numbers not provided; $P = 0.02$).

Harms: Adverse effects associated with imipramine treatment included blurred vision, tachycardia, palpitations, blood pressure changes, insomnia, nervousness, malaise, dizziness, headache, nausea, vomiting, and reduced appetite (see harms of prescription antidepressant drugs under depressive disorders, p 78).[14,17]

Panic disorder

Comment: The review included clomiprimine as a serotonin reuptake inhibitor. This drug is also often described as a tricyclic antidepressant.[13] The review used improvement as an outcome measure without a clear definition of this term. In the additional RCT and the second subsequent RCT, flexible dosing was used according to tolerance and therapeutic need.[14,15] In the subsequent RCT comparing imipramine versus placebo, relapse rate was not clearly defined.[16]

OPTION   **SELECTIVE SEROTONIN REUPTAKE INHIBITORS**

One systematic review and one subsequent RCT have found that selective serotonin reuptake inhibitors versus placebo improve symptoms in panic disorder.

Benefits: We found one systematic review (see benefits of tricyclic antidepressants, p 115 and benzodiazepines, p 117)[13] and one subsequent RCT.[18] The systematic review (search date not stated, 27 RCTs, 2348 people) found that selective serotonin reuptake inhibitors (paroxetine, fluvoxamine, zimelidine, and clomiprimine; see comment below) versus placebo significantly increased the number of people who improved ($P < 0.0001$; see comment below).[13] The subsequent RCT (279 people) compared five groups: oral citalopram (10 or 15 mg/day); oral citalopram (20 or 30 mg/day); oral citalopram (40 or 60 mg/day); oral clomiprimine (60 or 90 mg/day); and placebo.[18] It found that citalopram (at all doses) versus placebo significantly increased the number of people who responded (defined as no panic attacks and either no episodic increases in anxiety or only slight increases in anxiety precipitated by definite events or activities) after 12 months (citalopram 10 or 15 mg/day v placebo; $P = 0.05$; citalopram 20 or 30 mg/day v placebo; $P = 0.001$; citalopram 40 or 60 mg/day v placebo; $P = 0.003$; results presented graphically).

Harms: The subsequent RCT reported that harms associated with citalopram included headache, tremor, dry mouth, and somnolence (see harms of prescription antidepressant drugs under depressive disorders, p 78).[18]

Comment: The review included clomiprimine as a selective serotonin reuptake inhibitor, although this drug is often described as a tricyclic antidepressant.[13] In addition, the review used improvement as an outcome measure without clearly defining this term. In the subsequent RCT, 28/54 (52%) people completed the trial; analysis was by intention to treat and people who withdrew from the trial were counted as treatment failures.[18] The RCT used flexible dosing according to tolerance and therapeutic need. Selective serotonin reuptake inhibitors can cause initial increased anxiety, which can exacerbate a tendency to focus on internal sensations and to avoid situations that trigger these sensations (catastrophise somatic sensations). Education about this event is likely to improve adherence with medication.

We found no evidence on the long term effects of monoamine oxidase inhibitors in panic disorder.

Benefits: We found no systematic review and no RCTs.

Harms: We found no evidence of harms associated specifically with the use of monoamine oxidase inhibitors in the long term treatment of panic disorder.

Comment: Our search strategy excluded studies with follow up of less than 6 months.

Two RCTs found insufficient evidence on the effects of buspirone in people with panic disorder.

Benefits: We found no systematic review but found two RCTs.[19,20] The first RCT (48 people) compared oral buspirone (maximum 60 mg/day) plus cognitive behavioural therapy (see glossary, p 118) versus placebo plus cognitive behavioural therapy for 16 weeks.[19] It found that oral buspirone plus cognitive behavioural therapy significantly improved self rated panic and agoraphobia scores after 1 year (using a 90 point symptom scale where each symptom was graded from 0 = not present, to 4 = severe; P = 0.03; absolute numbers not provided). The second RCT (41 people with panic disorder and agoraphobia) compared 16 weeks of oral buspirone (30 mg/day) plus cognitive behavioural therapy versus 16 weeks of placebo plus cognitive behavioural therapy.[20] It found no significant difference in the number of people who had a reduction of at least 50% in their agoraphobic symptoms after 68 weeks (44% with buspirone plus cognitive behavioural therapy v 68% with placebo plus cognitive behavioural therapy; absolute numbers of people not provided).

Harms: The RCTs did not report harms (see harms of buspirone under generalised anxiety disorder, p 96).

Comment: The first RCT used a flexible dosing regimen with maximum dose adjustment according to tolerance and therapeutic need.[19]

One systematic review and one additional RCT have found that alprazolam reduces the numbers of panic attacks and improves symptoms in people with panic disorder. Benzodiazepines are associated with a wide range of adverse effects both during their use and after treatment has been withdrawn.

Benefits: We found one systematic review (search date not stated, 27 RCTs, 2348 people) (see benefits of tricyclic antidepressants, p 115 and SSRIs, p 116),[13] and one additional RCT.[14] The review found that alprazolam versus placebo significantly increased the number of people judged to have improved (P < 0.0001; see comment below).[13] The additional RCT (181 people with panic disorder with

Panic disorder

or without agoraphobia) compared three treatments: oral alprazolam (maximum 10 mg/day; see comment below), oral imipramine (maximum 225 mg/day; see comment below), and placebo (see benefits of tricyclic antidepressants, p 115 and SSRIs, p 909).[14] It found that alprazolam versus placebo was associated with fewer panic attacks after 8 months (results presented graphically; significance not calculated).[14]

Harms: The systematic review did not report harms.[13] Adverse effects associated with alprazolam include sedation, insomnia, memory lapses, nervousness, irritability, dry mouth, tremor, impaired coordination, constipation, urinary retention, altered libido, and altered appetite (see harms of benzodiazepines under generalised anxiety disorder, p 887).[14] We found one non-systematic review of the effects of benzodiazepines in anxiety disorder in people with a history of substance abuse or dependence.[21] The review reported that the mortality of long term benzodiazepine users was no higher than matched controls. It reported that the most pronounced adverse effects followed sudden withdrawal and included tinnitus, paraesthesias, vision disturbance, depersonalisation, seizures, withdrawal psychosis, and persistent discontinuation syndrome.

Comment: The review used improvement as an outcome measure without clearly defining this term.[13] The additional RCT used flexible dosing according to tolerance and therapeutic need.[14] Many RCTs of psychological and pharmacological treatments (even those not involving benzodiazepines) allowed people to receive small amounts of anxiolytic drugs during the study because benzodiazepine abuse is quite prevalent in people who suffer from panic disorder.

GLOSSARY

Cognitive behavioural therapy Brief structured treatment using relaxation and exposure procedures, and aimed at changing dysfunctional beliefs and negative automatic thoughts (typically 20 sessions over 12–16 wks).

REFERENCES

1. American Psychiatric Association. *Diagnostic and statistical manual of mental disorders*, 4th ed. Washington, DC: American Psychiatric Association, 1994.

2. World Health Organization. *The ICD-10 classification of mental and behavioural disorders*. Geneva: World Health Organization, 1992.

3. Robins LN, Regier DA, eds. *Psychiatric Disorders in America: The Epidemiologic Catchment Area Study*. New York, NY: The Free Press, 1991.

4. Weissman MM, Bland MB, Canino GJ, et al. The cross-national epidemiology of panic disorder. *Arch Gen Psychiatry* 1997;54:305–309.

5. Andrews G, Henderson S, Hall W. Prevalence, comorbidity, disability and service utilisation. Overview of the Australian National Mental Health Survey. *Br J Psychiatry* 2001;178: 145–153.

6. Last CG, Barlow DH, O'Brien GT. Precipitants of agoraphobia: role of stressful life events. *Psychol Rep* 1984;54:567–570.

7. De Loof C, Zandbergen H, Lousberg T, Pols H, Griez E. The role of life events in the onset of panic disorder. *Behav Res Ther* 1989;27: 461–463.

8. Rapee RM, Mattick RP, Murrell E. Impact of life events on subjects with panic disorder and on comparison subjects. *Am J Psychiatry* 1990;147: 640–644.

9. Hirschfield RMA. Panic disorder: Diagnosis, epidemiology and clinical course. *J Clin Psychiatry* 1996;57:3–8.

10. Andrews G, Creamer M, Crino R, Hunt C, Lampe L, Page A. *The Treatment of Anxiety Disorders*. Cambridge: Cambridge University Press, 1994.

11. Page AC, Andrews G. Do specific anxiety disorders show specific drug problems? *Aust N Z J Psychiatry* 1996;30:410–414.

12. Gorman JM, Coplan JD. Comorbidity of depression and panic disorder. *J Clin Psychiatry* 1996;57:34–41.

13. Boyer W. Serotonin uptake inhibitors are superior to imipramine and alprazolam in alleviating panic attacks: a meta-analysis. *Int Clin Psychopharmacol* 1995;10:45–49. Search date not stated; primary sources Medline, Embase, Psychlit, and sponsoring agencies of two trials contacted for supplementary statistical information.

14. Curtis GC, Massana J, Udina C, Ayuso JL, Cassano GB, Perugi G. Maintenance drug therapy of panic disorder. *J Psychiatr Res* 1993;27: 127–142.

15. Barlow DH, Gorman J, Shear MK, Woods SW. Cognitive-behavioral therapy, imipramine, or their combination for panic disorder: A randomized controlled trial [see comments]. *JAMA* 2000;283: 2529–2536.

16. Mavissakalian MR, Perel JM. Long-term maintenance and discontinuation of imipramine therapy in panic disorder with agoraphobia. *Arch Gen Psychiatry* 1999;56:821–827.

17. Cassano GB, Toni C, Petracca A, et al. Adverse effects associated with the short-term treatment of panic disorder with imipramine, alprazolam or placebo. *Eur Neuropsychopharmacol* 1994;4:47–53.

18. Lepola UM, Wade AG, Leinonen EV, et al. A controlled, prospective, 1-year trial of citalopram in the treatment of panic disorder. *J Clin Psychiatry* 1998;59:528–534.

19. Bouvard M, Mollard E, Guerin J, Cottraux J. Study and course of the psychological profile in 77 patients expressing panic disorder with agoraphobia after cognitive behaviour therapy with or without buspirone. *Psychother Psychosom* 1997;66:27–32.

20. Cottraux J, Note ID, Cungi C, et al. A controlled study of cognitive behaviour therapy with buspirone or placebo in panic disorder with agoraphobia. *Br J Psychiatry* 1995;167: 635–641.

21. Posternak M, Mueller T. Assessing the risks and benefits of benzodiazepines for anxiety disorders in patients with a history of substance abuse or dependence. *Am J Addict* 2001;10: 48–68.

Shailesh Kumar
Division of Psychiatry
Auckland Medical School
Auckland
New Zealand

Mark Oakley-Browne
Professor of Rural Psychiatry
Monash University
Gippsland Victoria
Australia

Competing interests: SK was reimbursed by Eli-Lilly, the manufacturers of Prozac (fluoxetine), to attend two psychiatric symposia. MOB has been paid by GlaxoSmithKline, the manufacturer of Aropax (paroxetine), for contributing to educational sessions for general practitioners. The programme topic was "The recognition and management of generalized anxiety disorder".

Search date May 2001

Jonathan Bisson

Key Messages

Prevention

■ One systematic review found no evidence that debriefing prevents post-traumatic stress disorder (PTSD). This systematic review included one RCT, which found that debriefing was associated with an increased risk of PTSD at 1 year.

■ We found limited evidence from three RCTs that multiple episode cognitive behavioural therapy or prolonged exposure therapy are of benefit in the prevention of PTSD. Two small RCTs have found that five sessions of either cognitive behavioural therapy or prolonged exposure therapy are superior to supportive counselling for preventing PTSD in people with acute stress disorder after a traumatic event. One RCT has found evidence of more benefit from one to six sessions of cognitive behavioural therapy than from standard care. One RCT found no evidence of benefit from multiple episode psychological intervention.

Treatment

- Evidence from mainly small RCTs suggests benefit from specific psychological treatments (cognitive behavioural therapy, eye movement desensitisation and reprocessing) compared with supportive counselling, relaxation therapy, or no treatment.

- One systematic review has found that sertraline reduces symptoms more than placebo. We found insufficient evidence on the effects of antipsychotic drugs or carbamazepine.

DEFINITION	PTSD occurs after a major traumatic event. Symptoms include upsetting thoughts and nightmares about the traumatic event, avoidance behaviour, numbing of general responsiveness, increased irritability, and hypervigilance.[1]
INCIDENCE/ PREVALENCE	One large cross sectional study in the USA found that 10% women and 20% men experience PTSD at some stage in their lives.[2]
AETIOLOGY/ RISK FACTORS	Risk factors include major trauma such as rape, a history of psychiatric disorders, acute distress and depression after the trauma, lack of social support, and personality factors (such as neuroticism).[3]
PROGNOSIS	One large cross sectional study in the USA found that over a third of sufferers continued to satisfy the criteria for a diagnosis of PTSD 6 years after diagnosis.[2] Cross sectional studies provide weak evidence about prognosis.
AIMS	To reduce initial distress after a traumatic event; to prevent PTSD and other psychiatric disorders; to reduce levels of distress in the long term; and to improve function and quality of life.
OUTCOMES	Presence or absence of PTSD and severity of symptoms. Scoring systems include impact of event scale and clinician administered PTSD scale.
METHODS	*Clinical Evidence* search and appraisal May 2001.

QUESTION   **What are the effects of preventive psychological interventions?**

One systematic review found no evidence that single episode interventions prevent PTSD. This systematic review included one RCT, which found that debriefing was associated with an increased risk of PTSD at 1 year. Three RCTs found limited evidence that cognitive behavioural therapy or prolonged exposure therapy can prevent PTSD. One RCT found no difference between multiple educational and psychological interventions versus no treatment in PTSD prevention rates at 6 months following a road traffic accident.

Benefits: **Single episode intervention:** We found one systematic review (search date not stated, 8 RCTs, 607 people) comparing early single episode interventions ("debriefing") versus no intervention.[4] The RCTs used psychological debriefing (see glossary, p 125) or similar techniques. The review found that more people treated with debriefing still had PTSD at 3–5 months but the difference was not significant (OR [3–5 months] 1.2, 95% CI 0.7 to 2.1; OR [12 months] 2.0, 95% CI 0.9 to 4.5). One of the RCTs followed people for 1 year after debriefing and found that debriefing versus no treatment was associated with increased rates of PTSD (OR 2.9, 95% CI 1.1 to 7.5). **Multiple episode intervention:** We found no systematic review. We found four RCTs. The first RCT (151 people) compared three to six sessions of educational and cognitive behavioural techniques with no psychological intervention.[5] Intervention began at least 1 month after a road traffic accident. There were no significant differences in rates of development of PTSD between groups at 6 months. The second RCT (24 people) compared five sessions of cognitive behavioural therapy (see glossary, p 125) versus five sessions of supportive counselling (see glossary, p 125) in people with acute stress disorder within 2 weeks of a road accident or industrial accident.[6] Cognitive behavioural therapy was associated with a large reduction in the number of people who met PTSD diagnostic criteria immediately after treatment (8% v 83% with supportive counselling; P < 0.001) and at 6 months (17% v 67% with supportive counselling; P < 0.05).[7] The third RCT (66 survivors of road accidents or non-sexual assault with acute stress disorder) evaluated five 90 minute sessions of prolonged exposure (see glossary, p 125) versus supportive counselling versus prolonged exposure plus anxiety management. Immediately after completion of treatment, significantly lower rates of PTSD were found in the prolonged exposure group (14%) and in the prolonged exposure plus anxiety management group (20%) compared with the supportive counselling group (56%). The differences were still significant at 6 months' follow up (15% v 23% v 67%).[8] The fourth RCT (132 French bus drivers who had been attacked)[9] compared one to six sessions of cognitive behavioural therapy with standard care. At 6 months' follow up, the reductions in anxiety and intrusive symptoms measures were significantly greater in the treatment group, but there were no significant differences in depression or avoidance symptom measures between the groups.

Harms: Two RCTs of single episode intervention included in the systematic review found an increased risk of subsequent psychological problems in people receiving the intervention. However, initial traumatic exposure had been higher in these people.[4]

Comment: The systematic review found that the overall quality of the RCTs was poor.[4] Problems included lack of blinding, failure to state loss to follow up, and lack of intention to treat analysis despite high withdrawal rates. These methodological problems are also apparent in the multiple episode intervention RCTs. The first multiple episode psychological treatment RCT[5] included multiple types of intervention (help, information, support, reality testing/confrontation) in the treatment group.

QUESTION   What are the effects of psychological treatments?

RCTs, mainly small, have found evidence of benefit from specific psychological treatments compared with supportive counselling, relaxation therapy, or no treatment.

Benefits: We found one systematic review of psychological treatments for PTSD (search date not stated, 17 RCTs, 690 people).[7] The RCTs compared a range of specific psychological treatments versus supportive counselling (see glossary, p 125) or no intervention. All trials found that psychological treatment was associated with a greater improvement in immediate outcome (using a composite score of PTSD symptoms, anxiety, and depression) compared with supportive counselling or no treatment (overall effect size immediately after treatment 0.54; 95% CI not provided). The difference was still evident at 1 year (overall effect size from 12 RCTs with long term follow up 0.53; CI not provided). **Cognitive behavioural therapy:** See glossary, p 125. We found one systematic review (search date not stated, 17 RCTs, 690 people)[7] and two subsequent RCTs.[10,11] The review identified 14 RCTs of cognitive behavioural therapy in people with PTSD. Although many were of poor quality, all described a positive effect compared with no treatment. One RCT (45 people) in the review evaluated three types of cognitive therapy and found that all were better than no treatment at 3 months (effect sizes compared with no treatment: stress inoculation 1.1, 95% CI 0.66 to 1.5; supportive counselling 0.55, 95% CI 0.17 to 0.94; prolonged exposure therapy 1.67, 95% CI 1.2 to 2.1).[12] One subsequent RCT (87 people) compared exposure, cognitive therapy, or both, with relaxation therapy (see glossary, p 125).[10] The trial found that all cognitive behavioural therapies reduced symptoms of PTSD more than relaxation therapy, immediately and at 3 months (53 people assessed; no intention to treat analysis performed).[13] The second subsequent RCT (54 people) found that 39% of people continued to suffer from PTSD 1 year after sixteen 1 hour sessions of imaginal exposure therapy or cognitive therapy. There was no difference in the prevalence of PTSD between the two treatment groups.[11] **Eye movement desensitisation and reprocessing (EMDR):** We found one systematic review (search date 1999, 16 RCTs, 563 people).[14] Two RCTs found EMDR (see glossary, p 125) was as effective as exposure therapy, three found that EMDR was more effective than relaxation therapy, and three found that EMDR was more effective than remaining on a waiting list. Five RCTs considered EMDR with and without eye movements. In two RCTs, eyes moving was more effective than eyes fixed. In three RCTs there was no difference. **Affect management:** We found one RCT (48 women) comparing 15 weeks of affect management (see glossary, p 125) treatment (as adjunctive therapy to drug treatment) versus waiting list control.[15] The RCT found that control of PTSD and dissociative symptoms were greater with affect management. **Other psychological treatments:** We found one RCT (112 people), which found no significant difference between psychodynamic psychotherapy (see glossary, p 125), exposure therapy, and hypnotherapy (see glossary, p 125). However, all were slightly better than remaining on the waiting list (no treatment control). The trial did not quantify results.[16] One RCT (42 police officers)[17] evaluated brief eclectic psychotherapy (which combines components of cognitive behavioural therapy and psychodynamic therapy) over 16 sessions of treatment. The treatment group fared better than a waiting list control after treatment (9% v 50% remained PTSD positive) and at 3 months' follow up (4% v 65% remained PTSD positive). **Inpatient treatment programme:** We found no RCTs. **Drama therapy:** See glossary, p 125. We found no RCTs.

Post-traumatic stress disorder

Harms: The RCTs gave no information of harms. Overall, cognitive behavioural therapy seems well tolerated. However, there have been case reports in some people of "imaginal flooding" (a form of cognitive behavioural therapy) worsening symptoms, leading to calls for caution when assessing people for treatment.[18] The RCT of affect management treatment had a high withdrawal rate (31%), specific drug treatments were not stated, and the analysis was not by intention to treat.

Comment: None.

QUESTION   What are the effects of drug treatments?

One systematic review found limited evidence that sertraline reduced symptoms more than placebo. We found insufficient evidence on the benefits of fluoxetine, brofaromine, amitriptyline, lamotrigine, benzodiazepines, antipsychotics, carbamazepine, imipramine, or phenelzine.

Benefits: We found one systematic review (search date 1999,[19] 15 RCTs, 9 with sufficient data for inclusion in the analysis, 868 people) of pharmacotherapy for PTSD, which used the Clinical Global Impressions scale change item or close equivalent as the primary outcome measure. The proportion of non-responders was lower in the pharmacotherapy group than the control group (RR 0.72, 95% CI 0.64 to 0.83). Two studies considered sertraline (42 people: OR 0.44, 95% CI 0.12 to 1.60; 183 people: OR 0.44, 95% CI 0.24 to 0.78), one paroxetine (280 people: OR 0.64, 95% CI 0.40 to 1.02), one fluoxetine (53 people: OR 0.30, 95% CI 0.09 to 1.02), two brofaromine (114 people: OR 0.94, 95% CI 0.45 to 1.99; 64 people: OR 0.40, 95% CI 0.15 to 1.08), one amitriptyline (40 people: OR 0.41, 95% CI 0.12 to 1.42), one lamotrigine (14 people: OR 0.39, 95% CI 0.04 to 3.71), one imipramine (41 people: OR 0.23, 95% CI 0.07 to 0.78), and one phenelzine (37 people: OR 0.21, 95% CI 0.06 to 0.73). **Antipsychotic drugs:** We found no systematic review and no RCTs. **Carbamazepine:** We found no systematic review and no RCTs. **Benzodiazepines:** We found no systematic review. One RCT was not included in the systematic review above because of insufficient data.

Harms: The trials gave no information about harms. Known adverse effects include possible hypertensive crisis with monoamine oxidase inhibitors (and also the need for dietary restriction), anticholinergic effects with tricyclic antidepressants, nausea and headache with SSRIs (see harms of prescription antidepressant drugs under depressive disorders, p 78) and dependency with benzodiazepines (see harms of benzodiazepines under generalised anxiety disorder, p 94).

Comment: Small trial sizes and different populations make it difficult to compare results. Other treatments or combinations of drug and psychological treatment await evaluation. It is difficult to interpret effect sizes in terms of clinical importance rather than statistical significance. Some categorise effect sizes of less than 0.5 as small; between 0.5 and 0.8 as medium; and greater than 0.8 as large.

GLOSSARY

Affect management A type of group treatment focusing on regulation of mood.

Cognitive behavioural therapy Covers a variety of techniques. *Imaginal exposure* entails exposure to a detailed account or image of what happened. *Real life exposure* involves confronting real life situations that have become associated with the trauma and cause fear and distress. *Cognitive therapy* entails challenging distorted thoughts about the trauma, the self, and the world. *Stress inoculation* entails instruction in coping skills and some cognitive techniques such as restructuring.

Drama therapy Entails using drama as a form of expression and communication.

Eye movement desensitisation and reprocessing (EMDR) Entails asking the person to focus on the traumatic event, a negative cognition associated with it, and the associated emotions.[20] The person is then asked to follow the therapist's finger as it moves from side to side.

Hypnotherapy Entails hypnosis to allow people to work through the traumatic event.

Prolonged exposure A type of cognitive behavioural treatment that includes repeated exposure to memories of the trauma, and to non-dangerous real life situations that are avoided because of trauma related fear.

Psychodynamic psychotherapy Entails analysis of defence mechanisms, interpretations, and pre-trauma experiences.

Psychological debriefing A technique that entails detailed consideration of the traumatic event and the normalisation of psychological reactions.

Relaxation therapy A technique involving imagination of relaxing situations to induce muscular and mental relaxation.

Supportive counselling A non-directive intervention dealing with current issues rather than the trauma itself.

REFERENCES

1. American Psychiatric Association. *Diagnostic and statistical manual of mental disorders*. 4th ed. Washington: APA, 1994.

2. Kessler RC, Sonnega A, Bromet E, et al. Posttraumatic stress disorder in the national comorbidity survey. *Arch Gen Psychiatry* 1995;52: 1048–1060.

3. O'Brien S. *Traumatic events and mental health*. Cambridge: Cambridge University Press, 1998.

4. Wessely S, Bisson J. Brief psychological interventions ("debriefing") for trauma-related symptoms and prevention of post traumatic stress disorder (Cochrane Review). In: The Cochrane Library, Issue 1, 2001. Oxford: Update Software. Search date not stated; primary sources Medline, Embase, Psychlit, Pilots Traumatic Stress Database, Biosis, Pascal, *Occup Health Saf*, CDSR, trials register of the Cochrane Depression, Anxiety and Neurosis Group, hand search of *J Trauma Stress*, and contact with experts.

5. Brom D, Kleber RJ, Hofman MC. Victims of traffic accidents: incidence and prevention of post-traumatic stress disorder. *J Clin Psychol* 1993;49: 131–140.

6. Bryant RA, Harvey AG, Basten C, Dang ST, Sackville T, Basten C. Treatment of acute stress disorder: a comparison of cognitive behavioural therapy and supportive counselling. *J Consult Clin Psychol* 1998;66:862–866.

7. Sherman JJ. Effects of psychotherapeutic treatments for PTSD: a meta-analysis of controlled clinical trials. *J Trauma Stress* 1998;11:413–436. Search date not stated; primary sources Psychlit, ERIC, Medline, Cinahl, Dissertation Abstracts, and Pilots Traumatic Stress Database.

8. Bryant RA, Sackville T, Dang ST, Moulds M, Guthrie R. Treating acute stress disorder: an evaluation of cognitive behavior therapy and supportive counselling techniques. *Am J Psychiatry* 1999;156:1780–1786.

9. Andre C, Lelord F, Legeron P, Reigner A, Delattre A. Controlled study of outcomes after 6 months to early intervention of bus driver victims of aggression [in French]. *Encephale* 1997;23: 65–71.

10. Rothbaum BO. A controlled study of eye movement desensitization and reprocessing in the treatment of posttraumatic stress disordered sexual assault victims. *Bull Menninger Clin* 1997; 61:317–334.

11. Tarrier N, Sommerfield C, Pilgrim H, Humphreys L. Cognitive therapy or imaginal exposure in the treatment of post-traumatic stress disorder. *Br J Psychiatry* 1999;175:571–575.

12. Foa EB, Rothbaum BO, Riggs DS, et al. Treatment of posttraumatic stress disorder in rape victims: a comparison between cognitive-behavioural procedures and counselling. *J Consult Clin Psychol* 1992;59:715–723.

13. Marks I, Lovell K, Noshirvani H, et al. Treatment of posttraumatic stress disorder by exposure and/or cognitive restructuring: a controlled study. *Arch Gen Psychiatry* 1998;55: 317–325.

14. Shepherd J, Stein K, Milne R. Eye movement desensitization and reprocessing in the treatment of post-traumatic stress disorder: a review of an emerging therapy. *Psychological Med* 2000;30: 863–871. Search date 1999; primary sources Medline, Embase, Healthstar, Psychlit, Cochrane

Post-traumatic stress disorder

Library, Best Evidence, National Research Register, the Medical Research Council trials database, Internet sites on PTSD, hand searches of reference lists, and personal contact with experts in the field.

15. Zlotnick C, Shea T, Rosen K, et al. An affect-management group for women with posttraumatic stress disorder and histories of childhood sexual abuse. *J Trauma Stress* 1997;10: 425–436.

16. Brom D, Kleber RJ, Defares PB. Brief psychotherapy of posttraumatic stress disorders. *J Consult Clin Psychol* 1989;57:607–612.

17. Gersons BPR, Carlier IVE, Lamberts RD, Van der Kolk BA. Randomised clinical trial of brief eclectic psychotherapy for police officers with posttraumatic stress disorder. *J Trauma Stress* 2000;13:333–348.

18. Pitman RK, Altman B, Greenwald E, et al. Psychiatric complications during flooding therapy for posttraumatic stress disorder. *J Clin Psychiatry* 1991;52:17–20.

19. Stein DJ, Zungu-Dirwayi N, Van der Linden GJ, Seedat S. Pharmacotherapy for Posttraumatic Stress Disorder (Cochrane Review). In: The Cochrane Library, Issue 1, 2001. Oxford: Update Software. Search date 1999; primary sources Medline, Psychlit, Pilots Traumatic Stress Database, Dissertation Abstracts, trials register of the Cochrane Depression, Anxiety and Neurosis Controlled Group, hand searches of reference lists, and personal contact with PTSD researchers and pharmaceutical companies.

20. Shapiro F. Eye movement desensitisation: a new treatment for post-traumatic stress disorder. *J Behav Ther Exp Psychiatry* 1989;20:211–217.

Jonathan Bisson
Consultant Liaison Psychiatrist
Cardiff and Vale NHS Trust
Cardiff
UK

Competing interests: None declared.

Key Messages

- Most evidence is from systematic reviews of RCTs that report different outcomes. There is a need for larger trials, over longer periods, with well designed end points, including standardised, validated symptom scales.

Systematic reviews have found that:

- Chlorpromazine and haloperidol improve clinical outcomes compared with placebo, but are associated with more adverse effects.

- There is limited evidence of benefit from depot haloperidol decanoate compared with placebo.

Schizophrenia

- The newer antipsychotic drugs loxapine, molindone, pimozide, amisulpride, olanzapine, quetiapine, risperidone, sulpiride, thioridazine, ziprasidone, and zotepine are as effective as standard antipsychotics and have different profiles of adverse effects.

- Clozapine is more effective than standard antipsychotics but is associated with potentially fatal blood dyscrasias.

- Relapse rates are significantly reduced by continuing antipsychotic medication for at least 6 months after an acute episode, by family interventions, and by psychoeducational interventions. Weaker evidence suggests that social skills training and cognitive behavioural therapy may also reduce relapse rates.

- No intervention has been consistently found to reduce negative symptoms.

RCTs have found:

- Limited evidence that compliance therapy, behavioural therapy, and psychoeducational therapy may improve adherence with antipsychotic medication. One systematic review has found that family therapy is unlikely to improve adherence.

DEFINITION	Schizophrenia is characterised by the "positive symptoms" (see glossary, p 148) of auditory hallucinations, delusions, and thought disorder, and the "negative symptoms" (see glossary, p 148) of demotivation, self neglect, and reduced emotion.[1]
INCIDENCE/ PREVALENCE	Onset of symptoms typically occurs in early adult life (average age 25 years) and is earlier in men than women. Prevalence worldwide is 2–4/1000. One in 100 people will develop schizophrenia in their lifetime.[2,3]
AETIOLOGY/ RISK FACTORS	Risk factors include a family history (although no major genes have been identified); obstetric complications; developmental difficulties; central nervous system infections in childhood; cannabis use; and acute life events.[2] The precise contributions of these factors and ways in which they may interact are unclear.
PROGNOSIS	About three quarters of people suffer recurrent relapse and continued disability, although outcomes were worse in the pretreatment era.[4] Outcome may be worse in people with insidious onset and delayed initial treatment, social isolation, or a strong family history; in people living in industrialised countries; in men; and in people who misuse drugs.[3] Drug treatment is generally successful in treating positive symptoms, but up to a third of people derive little benefit and negative symptoms are notoriously difficult to treat. About half of people with schizophrenia do not adhere to treatment in the short term. The figure is even higher in the longer term.[5]
AIMS	To relieve symptoms and to improve quality of life, with minimal adverse effects of treatment.
OUTCOMES	Severity of positive and negative symptoms; global clinical improvement; global clinical impression (a composite measure of symptoms and everyday functioning); rate of relapse; adherence to treatment; adverse effects of treatment.
METHODS	Clinical Evidence search and appraisal August 2001. Most of the trials we found were small, short term, with high withdrawal rates, and many different outcome measures.[6] There were a large number of high quality recent systematic reviews. Therefore, if possible, we

focused primarily on systematic reviews at the expense of subsequent RCTs and included only the outcomes we thought were the most clinically relevant (because different treatments are associated with different benefits and harms, we used estimates of global effectiveness if they were available). We searched for placebo controlled studies for standard antipsychotic medication and comparative studies for newer antipsychotics.

QUESTION | **What are the effects of drug treatments?**

OPTION | **CHLORPROMAZINE**

One systematic review has found that chlorpromazine produces global improvement in the short and medium term compared with placebo, but adverse effects make it unacceptable to many people.

Benefits:
Versus placebo: We found one systematic review (search date 1999, 45 RCTs, 3116 people, mean dose 511 mg/day, range 25–2000 mg/day).[7] Chlorpromazine was more effective than placebo. Chlorpromazine significantly reduced the proportion of people at 6 months who had no improvement on a psychiatrist rated global impression scale (583/921 [63%] with chlorpromazine v 609/790 [77%] with placebo; RR 0.76, 95% CI 0.71 to 0.80; NNT 7, 95% CI 5 to 10) and significantly reduced the proportion of people at 6 months who had marked or worse severity of illness on a psychiatrist rated scale (323/493 [66%] with chlorpromazine v 231/285 [81%] with placebo; RR 0.77, 95% CI 0.71 to 0.84; NNT 5, 95% CI 4 to 8).[7]

Harms:
Versus placebo: The systematic review found that chlorpromazine caused significantly higher rates of sedation (RR 2.4, 95% CI 1.7 to 3.3; NNH 6, 95% CI 4 to 8), acute dystonias (RR 3.1, 95% CI 1.3 to 7.6; NNH 24, 95% CI 14 to 77), parkinsonism (RR 2.6, 95% CI 1.2 to 5.4; NNH 10, 95% CI 8 to 16), weight gain (RR 4.4, 95% CI 2.1 to 9; NNH 3, 95% CI 2 to 5), skin photosensitivity (RR 5.2, 95% CI 3 to 10; NNH 7, 95% CI 6 to 10), dizziness caused by hypotension (RR 1.9, 95% CI 1.3 to 2.6; NNH 12, 95% CI 8 to 20), and dry mouth (RR 4, 95% CI 1.6 to 10; NNH 19, 95% CI 12 to 37).[7] Chlorpromazine was also associated with a non-significantly higher rate of seizures (RR 2.4, 95% CI 0.4 to 16) and blood dyscrasias (RR 2.0, 95% CI 0.7 to 6). We found no long term data on the risk of tardive dyskinesia or the rare but potentially fatal neuroleptic malignant syndrome. Despite the frequent adverse effects, people receiving active treatment were more likely to stay in trials than those receiving placebo in both the short and the medium term.

Comment:
The review did not categorise symptoms as positive or negative as this information was rarely available from included trials. Relative risks and numbers needed to treat were based on 6 months' data. There was significant heterogeneity of the benefits results from the RCTs, but the analyses remained significant after removal of the heterogenous RCTs.[7]

OPTION   HALOPERIDOL

One systematic review has found that haloperidol versus placebo produces global improvement in the short term, but is associated with unpleasant extra-pyramidal adverse effects.

Benefits: **Versus placebo:** We found one systematic review (search date 1998, 20 RCTs, 1001 people).[8] Haloperidol (over a wide range of doses) was more effective than placebo for achieving psychiatrist rated marked global improvement after 6 weeks (3 RCTs: RR for global improvement with haloperidol v placebo 2.3, 95% CI 1.7 to 3.3; NNT 3, 95% CI 2 to 5), and after 24 months (8 RCTs: RR 1.5, 95% CI 1.2 to 1.7; NNT 3, 95% CI 3 to 5).

Harms: **Versus placebo:** The systematic review found that, compared with placebo, haloperidol was associated with significantly higher risk of acute dystonia (2 RCTs: RR 4.7, 95% CI 1.7 to 44; NNH 5, 95% CI 3 to 9), akathisia (3 RCTs: R 6.5, 95% CI 1.5 to 28; NNH 6, 95%CI 4 to 14), and parkinsonism (4 RCTs: R 8.9, 95% CI 2.6 to 31; NNH 3, 95% CI 2 to 5).[8] People taking haloperidol were more likely to be treated with anticholinergic drugs than those taking placebo (4 RCTs: R 4.9, 95% CI 1.01 to 24; NNH 2, 95%CI 1 to 3).

Comment: The median study size was 38 people, but the quality of the RCTs was higher than average for schizophrenia trials. Although the dose range was very wide, most studies used 4–20 mg day and adjusted dose according to need. The review found evidence of publication bias for the 6–24 months global outcome ratings.[8]

OPTION   THIORIDAZINE

One systematic review found limited evidence favouring thioridazine over placebo. It found no significant differences between thioridazine and standard antipsychotic medication, although thioridazine was less likely to cause symptoms of drug induced parkinsonism.

Benefits: We found one systematic review (search date 1999, 11 RCTs, 560 people).[9] **Versus placebo:** The review found no significant difference between thioridazine versus placebo for improvement in global mental state (RR 0.66, 95% CI 0.35 to 1.23). Two RCTs (65 people) found that thioridazine versus placebo improved global mental state at 6 months (RR for improved global mental state for placebo v thioridazine 0.34, 95% CI 0.21 to 0.56; NNT 2, 95% CI 1 to 6). Three short term trials found no significant differences between thioridazine and placebo in global mental state improvement. **Versus standard antipsychotic drugs:** The review (26 RCTs, 2397 people) found no significant difference between thioridazine versus standard antipsychotic medication in the risk of "being better or no worse" on clinical global impression, or in mental state improvements.[9]

Harms: **Versus placebo:** The review found no significant differences in adverse events.[9] **Versus standard antipsychotic drugs:** The review found one RCT (74 people) comparing thioridazine versus chlorpromazine, which found that thioridazine caused more cardio-vascular adverse events at 3 months (RR 3.2, 95% CI 1.4 to 7.0;

NNH 3, 95% CI 2 to 7), although by 6 months the difference was not statistically significant. The review found that thioridazine caused fewer extrapyramidal adverse events (1082 people: RR 0.48, 95% CI 0.28 to 0.81) and parkinsonism (340 people: RR 0.29, 95% CI 0.12 to 0.70).[9]

Comment: We found limited data on retinopathy and RCTs were generally short.

OPTION **DEPOT HALOPERIDOL DECANOATE**

One systematic review found limited evidence that depot haloperidol decanoate is more effective than placebo.

Benefits: **Versus placebo:** We found one systematic review (search date 1998, 2 RCTs, 78 people).[10] Both RCTs found that people taking depot haloperidol were more likely to stay in the RCT (OR 11, 95% CI 5 to 33; NNT 2, 95% CI 1 to 3). One RCT (22 people) comparing intramuscular depot haloperidol decanoate (mean dose 150 mg monthly) versus placebo found that haloperidol decanoate was more likely to result in a "reduced need for medication" at 4 months (RR 2.6, 95% CI 1.1 to 5.6; NNT with 4 months' treatment 2, 95% CI 1 to 2).

Harms: Fewer people receiving haloperidol versus placebo left the trial early (RR 0.2, 95% CI 0.1 to 0.4; NNT 2, 95% CI 1 to 3).[10]

Comment: The trial did not report how "reduced need for medication" was measured. Depot injection is believed to ensure adherence, but we found no evidence to support this belief.

OPTION **DEPOT PIPOTIAZINE PALMITATE**

One systematic review found limited evidence from two RCTs of no significant difference between depot pipotiazine (pipothiazine) palmitate and standard antipsychotic drugs.

Benefits: **Versus standard oral antipsychotic drugs:** We found one systematic review (search date 1998), which identified two RCTs, both conducted in the 1970s, comparing intramuscular pipotiazine palmitate versus normal treatment ("standard" oral antipsychotic drugs, chosen by physicians).[11] Neither found a significant difference between active treatment and control groups (first trial, 124 people: WMD in composite rating of psychotic symptoms at 18 months –3.1, 95% CI –7.3 to +1.2; second trial, 48 people: no quantified results provided).

Harms: **Versus standard oral antipsychotic drugs:** One RCT (mean dose 90 mg monthly) found that the number of people needing to take anticholinergic drugs for unspecified reasons was not significantly different between depot versus standard drugs (RR 0.9, 95% CI 0.7 to 1.1).[11] Meta-analysis combining both trials (mean dose 113 mg monthly for 6 months) found no overall difference in the numbers of people leaving the trial early (25% in both groups, RR 1.0, 95% CI 0.5 to 1.9).

Comment: Several other depot preparations are commercially available in different countries, but we found even less evidence for their efficacy versus placebo or standard antipsychotic drugs.

OPTION   LOXAPINE

One systematic review comparing loxapine and standard antipsychotic drugs found no significant difference in benefits or harms.

Benefits: **Versus standard antipsychotic drugs:** We found one systematic review (search date 1999, 22 RCTs, 1073 people), which compared loxapine (dose range 25–250 mg daily) versus standard antipsychotic drugs, usually chlorpromazine.[12] It found no significant differences in global improvement (9 RCTs, 411 people: RR of no improvement 0.9, 95% CI 0.7 to 1.2).

Harms: The systematic review found no significant difference in adverse effects.[12]

Comment: All RCTs were conducted in the USA or India and none lasted longer than 12 weeks.

OPTION   MOLINDONE

One systematic review found no significant difference between molindone and standard antipsychotic drugs in benefits or harms, but the trials were short and of poor quality.

Benefits: **Versus standard antipsychotic drugs:** We found one systematic review of molindone versus standard antipsychotic drugs (search date 1999, 13 controlled trials, 469 people).[13] It found no significant differences in global efficacy between molindone and standard antipsychotic drugs (4 RCTs, 150 people: RR no improvement 1.1, 95% CI 0.7 to 1.8).

Harms: No significant differences were found between molindone and standard antipsychotic drugs in total numbers of adverse events. One trial found that the rate of confusion was higher in people taking molindone (RR 3.2, 95% CI 1.4 to 7.3). There were no significant differences in the rates of movement disorders between molindone and standard antipsychotic drugs. Weight loss was more frequent in those taking molindone (2 RCTs, 60 people: RR 2.8, 95% CI 1.1 to 7.0). Molindone was associated with less frequent weight gain than standard antipsychotic drugs (2 RCTs, 60 people: RR 0.4, 95% CI 0.1 to 1.0).[13]

Comment: The RCTs in the review had methodological problems (in 4 trials it was unclear whether randomisation had been performed, 7 trials included people whose diagnosis was not operationally defined), and were brief (all lasted under 13 wks). We found no reliable evidence comparing molindone with either placebo or new antipsychotic drugs.

OPTION   PIMOZIDE

We found insufficient evidence from RCTs comparing pimozide versus placebo. One systematic review comparing pimozide versus standard antipsychotic drugs found no significant differences in benefits or harms.

Benefits: **Versus placebo:** We found one systematic review (search date 1999, 3 RCTs, 86 people) of pimozide versus placebo.[14] One RCT (20 people) found no significant difference in clinical global impression at 3 months. Two further small RCTs (66 people) found greater improvement at 6 months with pimozide, the significance of which depend on the statistical method used. **Versus standard antipsychotic drugs:** We found one systematic review (search date 1999, 1155 people) of pimozide (mean dose 7.5 mg daily, range 1–75 mg daily) versus a variety of standard antipsychotic drugs.[14] It found no significant differences in clinical global impression rates (3 RCTs, 206 people: RR 0.9, 95% CI 0.8 to 1.1).

Harms: **Versus placebo:** One small short RCT found more electrocardiograph changes in the pimozide group (T wave changes, RR 5, 95% CI 0.3 to 93). Doses used were on a sliding scale up to 40 mg daily. **Versus standard antipsychotic drugs:** Pimozide caused less sedation than standard antipsychotic drugs alone (RR 0.4, 95% CI 0.2 to 0.7; NNT 6, 95% CI 4 to 16), but was more likely to cause tremor (RR 1.6, 95 CI 1.1 to 2.3; NNH 6, 95% CI 3 to 44). There was no overall difference in cardiovascular symptoms such as rise or fall in blood pressure and dizziness between pimozide and other drugs. There was little usable electrocardiogram (ECG) data. One RCT in the review found no difference in ECG changes (RR 0.67, 95 CI 0.1 to 3.7).

Comment: Sudden death has been reported in a number of people taking pimozide at doses over 20 mg daily, but we found no evidence that pimozide is more likely to cause sudden death than other antipsychotic drugs. The manufacturer recommends periodic ECG monitoring in all people taking more than 16 mg daily of pimozide and avoidance of other drugs known to prolong the QT interval on an ECG or cause electrolyte disturbances (other antipsychotics, antihistamines, antidepressants, and diuretics). The trials comparing pimozide versus placebo may be too small to detect a clinically significant difference.

OPTION	POLYUNSATURATED FATTY ACIDS

One systematic review found limited evidence that polyunsaturated fatty acids compared with placebo reduced the subsequent use of antipsychotic medication.

Benefits: **Versus placebo:** We found one systematic review (search date 2000, 1 RCT, 30 people) of fatty acid supplementation versus placebo.[15] It found less need at 12 weeks for subsequent antipsychotic medication in those receiving fish oil compared with those receiving placebo (RR 0.6, 95% CI 0.4 to 0.9). The review also found a slight difference in average symptom severity scores favouring fish oil (26 people: WMD –13, 95% CI –22 to –3).

Harms: The RCT did not find significant adverse events.

Comment: The single relevant RCT cited in the systematic review is an unpublished conference proceeding. Other RCTs considered only augmentation of antipsychotic treatment.

OPTION   SULPIRIDE

One systematic review of 18 RCTs found no significant difference in benefits between sulpiride and other antipsychotic medication.

Benefits: We found one systematic review (search date 1998, 3 RCTs, 141 people).[16] **Versus placebo:** The review found that sulpiride was better than placebo for mental state but meta-analysis was not possible. **Versus standard antipsychotic drugs:** The review (13 RCTs, 97 people) found no significant differences in global improvement versus standard antipsychotic drugs (RR of not improved 0.96, 95% CI 0.90 to 1.02). Evidence on mental state was inadequate.[16]

Harms: **Versus placebo:** Limited adverse event data were reported.[16] No differences were found between sulpiride versus placebo for involuntary movements or hypersalivation. **Versus standard antipsychotic drugs:** The use of antiparkinson drugs was less frequent in the sulpiride group (RR 0.73, 95% CI 0.59 to 0.90).[16]

Comment: Trial quality was generally poor. Observational evidence and clinical experience suggest galactorrhoea may be a real problem, but trial data did not quantify the risk of occurrence.[17]

OPTION   AMISULPRIDE

One systematic review found limited evidence that amisulpride may be more effective than conventional antipsychotic drugs, although effects may be attributable to differences in dose. The review found that movement disorders were less likely compared with conventional antipsychotic drugs. One included RCT has found no evidence that amisulpride improved symptom scores more than risperidone.

Benefits: **Versus conventional antipsychotics:** We found no systematic review comparing amisulpride versus conventional antipsychotics. However, one systematic review (search date 1998, 683 people, trial duration 4–6 weeks) compared conventional antipsychotics versus atypical antipsychotics.[18] The review included four RCTs comparing amisulpride with conventional antipsychotics, usually haloperidol. Allocation concealment was unclear in all included trials. Overall, symptom reduction was greater with amisulpride than conventional antipsychotics (standardised effect size –0.35, 95% CI –0.52 to –0.18, indicating that about 64% [95% CI 57 to 70] of people do worse with conventional antipsychotics compared with amisulpride). **Versus other atypical antipsychotics:** The review identified one RCT comparing amisulpride versus risperidone (228 people, 8 weeks' duration), which found no significant differences between the two drugs in terms of the brief psychiatric rating scale total symptom scores.[18]

Harms: **Versus conventional antipsychotics:** Drop out rates were significantly lower with amisulpride than with conventional antipsychotics (NNT 9, 95% CI 5 to 22). Movement disorders, measured by the Simpson Angus scale, were less frequent with amisulpride compared with conventional antipsychotics (SMD –0.44, 95% CI –0.26

to −0.61). **Versus other atypical antipsychotics**: The RCT comparing amisulpride versus risperidone found no significant differences for adverse effects, extrapyramidal symptoms, or drop out rate.

Comment: All four short term RCTs included people randomised to relatively high doses of amisulpride (estimated equivalent to 20 mg haloperidol), which may have exaggerated results in favour of amisulpride. Meta-regression analysis found that, after adjustment for dose differences, atypical antipsychotics lose their therapeutic advantage over conventional antipsychotics, but remain superior for extrapyramidal adverse effects. Meta-regression was not available for amisulpride alone.[18]

| OPTION | OLANZAPINE |

Three systematic reviews found limited evidence that olanzapine may be more effective than standard antipsychotic drugs and good evidence that olanzapine has fewer adverse effects. Four systematic reviews found no evidence that olanzapine is more effective than other new antipsychotic drugs.

Benefits: We found five systematic reviews[18–22] and one subsequent RCT.[23] Three systematic reviews compared olanzapine versus standard antipsychotics[18–20] and four compared olanzapine versus other new antipsychotics.[18,20-22] **Versus standard antipsychotic drugs:** The first systematic review (search date 1999, 15 RCTs, 3282 people) compared olanzapine with standard antipsychotic drugs, usually haloperidol.[19] It found that olanzapine (2.5–25 mg daily) did not significantly reduce psychotic symptoms over 6–8 weeks compared with standard antipsychotic drugs (2778 people: RR for no important response, defined as a 40% reduction on any scale 0.9, 95% CI 0.76 to 1.06). The second systematic review (search date 1999, 4 RCTs, 2914 people) found that olanzapine was associated with slightly greater treatment success than haloperidol on a composite measure of positive and negative symptoms.[20] The third systematic review (search date 1998, 4 RCTs) similarly found that olanzapine improved symptoms compared with standard antipsychotics (WMD −0.22, 95% CI −0.30 to −0.14) indicating that 59% of people taking antipsychotics had poorer symptom score than people taking olanzapine. However, after adjustment for treatment doses, no significant benefit was found (see comment on amisulpride, p 135).[18] **Versus risperidone:** We found limited and conflicting evidence. Two systematic reviews (search date 1999, 1 RCT;[20] search date 1998, 2 RCTs[18]) and one subsequent RCT[23] found no significant difference between olanzapine and risperidone (results from first systematic review; RR for no clinically important response after 8 wks 0.93, 95% CI 0.85 to 1.01).[20] However, one further systematic review (search date 1999, 3 RCTs) found that olanzapine reduced symptom severity in the medium term, although it found no significant difference in the long term (at medium term follow up in 392 participants, composite symptom scores improved by 7.5 points with olanzapine v risperidone on a 210 point scale, 95% CI 2.9 to 12.0).[22] **Versus clozapine:** One systematic review (search date 1998, 1 RCT, 180 people) comparing olanzapine versus clozapine found no significant difference for clinical response rates (RR for no important clinical response 0.7, 95% CI 0.5 to 1.1).[21]

Harms: **Versus standard antipsychotic drugs:** Olanzapine versus standard antipsychotic drugs did not significantly reduce the number of people who withdrew from the trials at 6–8 weeks (36% v 49%; RR 0.9, 95% CI 0.7 to 1.1) or at 1 year (83% v 90%; OR 0.9, 95% CI 0.86 to 1.02).[19] Olanzapine versus standard antipsychotic drugs caused fewer extrapyramidal adverse effects (in heterogeneous data prone to bias), less nausea (2347 people; RR 0.7, 95% CI 0.6 to 0.9; NNT 25, 95% CI 14 to 85), vomiting (1996 people: RR 0.6, 95% CI 0.4 to 0.8; NNT 20, 95% CI 12 to 46), or drowsiness (2347 people: RR 0.8, 95% CI 0.7 to 0.9) than standard antipsychotic drugs.[19] Olanzapine was associated with a greater increase in appetite (1996 people: RR 1.7, 95% CI 1.4 to 2.0; NNH 10, 95% CI 7 to 15), and weight gain (heterogeneous data) than standard antipsychotic drugs.[19] The third systematic review found that drop out rate was lower with olanzapine than with haloperidol The difference in drop out rate did not persist after adjustment for dose.[18] Dystonia and akathisia were less frequent with olanzapine than haloperidol, even after adjustment for dose (ARR for dystonia with olanzapine v haloperidol 14%, 95% CI 11% to 17%; ARR for akathisia with olanzapine v haloperidol 4.8%, 95% CI 3.1% to 6.5%). Olanzapine was associated with a 12% (95% CI 8% to 15%) increase in excessive appetite compared with haloperidol.[18] **Versus risperidone:** The first systematic review (search date 1999, 1 RCT, 84 people) found that olanzapine compared with risperidone was associated with fewer extrapyramidal adverse effects (NNT to avoid causing 1 adverse effect 8), less parkinsonism (NNT 11), and less need for anticholinergic medication (NNT 8), but olanzapine caused more dry mouth (NNH 9), and greater weight gain (NNH 11).[19] One additional review found that risperidone was associated with a higher drop out rate than olanzapine (RR for drop out with risperidone v olanzapine 1.3, 95% CI 1.1 to 1.6).[22] One subsequent RCT (377 people) comparing olanzapine and risperidone found no significant differences for severity of extrapyramidal adverse effects, need for anticholinergics, or for drop out rate. Fewer people on risperidone experienced weight gain (AR for ≥ 7% weight gain 27.3% with olanzapine, 11.6% with risperidone).[23] **Versus clozapine:** One RCT (search date 1999, 180 people) found that olanzapine was associated with less nausea than clozapine (RR 0.1, 95% CI 0.01 to 0.8), but found no significant difference for movement disorders (RR for self reported symptoms of movement disorder 0.4, 95% CI 0.1 to 1.4).[21]

Comment: The results of the reviews are dominated by one large multicentre RCT reported by drug company employees. Benefits seem to be maximal at a dose of 15 mg daily, and higher doses may be associated with more harms. Results depended on the precise statistical test used. Reliability of results may be compromised by heterogeneity. Comparative trials of new antipsychotics tended to favour the treatment manufactured by the trial sponsor.

OPTION **QUETIAPINE**

Three systematic reviews comparing quetiapine with standard antipsychotic drugs found no significant differences in benefits, but significant reduction of some harms.

Benefits: **Versus standard antipsychotic drugs:** We found three systematic reviews.[18,20,24] The first review (search date 1999, 6 RCTs, 1414 people) identified two RCTs (809 people) comparing quetiapine with haloperidol and found no evidence of a difference in effectiveness on a composite measure of positive and negative symptoms.[20] The second review (search date 2000, 7 RCTs) of quetiapine (50–800 mg daily) versus standard antipsychotic drugs (usually haloperidol) found no significant differences in global improvement (1247 people: RR no important improvement in mental state 0.93, 95% CI 0.83 to 1.04).[24] The third review (search date 1998, 2 RCTs) also found no difference in overall symptom score (WMD –0.03, 95% CI –0.23 to +0.18).[18]

Harms: **Versus standard antipsychotic drugs:** The second review found quetiapine versus standard antipsychotic drugs was associated with fewer people leaving trials early (RR 0.87, 95% CI 0.76 to 0.99), less dystonia (RR 0.14, 95% CI 0.04 to 0.49), less akathisia (RR 0.24, 95% CI 0.15 to 0.38), and less parkinsonism (RR 0.22, 95% CI 0.15 to 0.33), but more dry mouth (RR 2.85, 95% CI 1.46 to 5.57).[24] The third systematic review found no difference between quetiapine and standard antipsychotic drugs for drop out rate (OR 0.70, 95% CI 0.46 to 1.06). Meta-regression analysis, which controlled for dose differences, found that as a group, new antipsychotic drugs reduced extrapyramidal adverse effects compared with standard drugs (see comment on amisulpiride, p 135).[18]

Comment: The evidence comes from a small number of short term trials that had substantial withdrawal rates and did not conduct intention to treat analyses.

OPTION **RISPERIDONE**

Three systematic reviews comparing risperidone versus standard antipsychotic drugs (mainly haloperidol) found limited evidence that risperidone may be more effective than standard antipsychotic drugs and good evidence that, at lower doses, risperidone has fewer adverse effects. Three systematic reviews found no significant difference between risperidone versus new antipsychotic drugs.

Benefits: **Versus standard antipsychotic drugs:** We found three systematic reviews[20,25,19] and one additional RCT.[26] The systematic reviews found that risperidone was more effective than haloperidol. The first systematic review (search date 1997, 14 RCTs, 3401 people) found that, at 12 weeks, risperidone (mean daily dose range 6.1–12 mg) was more effective than standard antipsychotic drugs, usually haloperidol.[25] Outcome was "clinical improvement", variably defined but usually a 20% reduction in general symptoms (2171 people: 11 RCTs; RR no improvement 0.8, 95% CI 0.7 to 0.9; NNT 10, 95% CI 7 to 16). No benefit was observed for the outcome of global clinical impression. The second systematic review (search date 1999, 9 RCTs, 2215 people) found that risperidone was associated with slightly greater success than haloperidol on a composite measure of positive and negative symptoms.[20] The third systematic review (search date 1998, 8 RCTs) found significant heterogeneity among six short term trials. Two long term trials found that risperidone improved symptom scores compared with standard antipsychotics (WMD −0.40, 95% CI −0.27 to −0.54 indicating that about 66% of people taking standard antipsychotics had worse composite symptom scores than with risperidone). However, this difference did not persist after controlling for dose of standard drug (see benefits of amisulpride, p 134).[18] The additional RCT (99 people) comparing a range of doses of risperidone with haloperidol found no overall significant difference in global outcome.[26] **Versus other new antipsychotic drugs:** See benefits of olanzapine, p 135. We found three systematic reviews,[18,21,22] which found no significant difference between risperidone versus clozapine (5 RCTs) or versus amisulpride (1 RCT) for outcomes including improvement in mental state. However, the RCTs were small and short, with high withdrawal rates. The third review found no difference in pooled efficacy in two trials comparing risperidone and clozapine.[18]

Harms:
Versus standard antipsychotic drugs: The first systematic review found that risperidone versus standard antipsychotic drugs caused no significant change in the number of people who withdrew from treatment (2166 people: RR 0.8, 95% CI 0.6 to 1.1). People taking risperidone developed fewer extrapyramidal effects (2279 people: RR 0.6, 95% CI 0.5 to 0.7; NNT 5, 95% CI 5 to 10), required less antiparkinsonian medication (2436 people: RR 0.6, 95% CI 0.5 to 0.7; NNT 7, 95% CI 5 to 10), and were less likely to develop daytime somnolence (2098 people: RR 0.9, 95% CI 0.7 to 0.99; NNT 22, 95% CI 11 to 500). Risperidone was associated with greater weight gain (1652 people: RR 1.4, 95% CI 1.1 to 1.7; NNH 13, 95% CI 8 to 36).[25] The additional RCT found no overall significant difference in the rate of adverse effects between risperidone and haloperidol.[26] The third systematic review found no difference for drop out rate between risperidone and haloperidol, but found that risperidone reduced symptoms of dystonia (WMD −0.26, 95% CI −0.39 to −0.12), parkinsonism (WMD −0.39, 95% CI −0.51 to −0.27), and dyskinesia (WMD −0.16, 95% CI −0.28 to −0.04) compared with haloperidol. Differences persisted after controlling for dose.[18]
Versus other new antipsychotic drugs: See harms of olanzapine, p 136. We found three systematic reviews,[18,21,22] which found no significant difference between risperidone and clozapine. The second systematic review (search date 1999, 1 RCT, 228 people) found amisulpride versus risperidone caused less agitation (RR 0.29, 95% CI 0.1 to 0.86), and less constipation (RR 0.13, 95% CI 0.2 to 1.0).[22]

Comment:
The reported benefits in the first review over standard antipsychotic drugs were marginal, and it found evidence of publication bias.[25] Sensitivity analyses found that benefits in clinical improvement and continuing treatment of risperidone compared with standard antipsychotic drugs were no longer significant if trials using more than 10 mg haloperidol daily were excluded.[25] This loss of significance

could be because of loss of power when trials were excluded. Exclusion of the higher dosage trials did not remove the difference in rate of extrapyramidal adverse effects.[25]

OPTION ZIPRASIDONE

One systematic review comparing ziprasidone with standard antipsychotic drugs found no significant difference in mental state improvement but did find a different profile of adverse effects.

Benefits: We found one systematic review (search date 1999, 7 RCTs, 824 people).[27] **Versus standard antipsychotics:** It identified four RCTs of ziprasidone versus standard antipsychotic drugs. It found no significant differences in mental state improvement in different trials (301 people: RR no important improvement in mental state 0.9, 95% CI 0.7 to 1.0).

Harms: **Versus standard antipsychotics:** The review found no clear difference in total adverse events between ziprasidone and haloperidol.[21] Ziprasidone was less likely to cause akathisia in the short term (438 people: RR 0.3, 95% CI 0.2 to 0.6; NNT 8, 95% CI 5 to 18), and in the long term (301 people: RR 0.3, 95% CI 0.1 to 0.7; NNT 9, 95% CI 5 to 21), and less likely to cause acute dystonia (438 people: RR 0.4, 95% CI 0.2 to 0.9; NNT 16, 95% CI 9 to 166). Ziprasidone was more likely to produce nausea and vomiting in both the short term (306 people: RR 3.6, 95% CI 1.8 to 7; NNT 5, 95% CI 4 to 8), and in the long term (301 people: RR 2.1, 95% CI 1 to 4; NNT 9, 95% CI 5 to 33). Intramuscular ziprasidone was significantly more likely to be associated with injection site pain than haloperidol (306 people: RR 5.3, 95% CI 1.3 to 22; NNT 12, 95% CI 7 to 27).

Comment: The duration of RCTs was less than 6 weeks. Most reported a withdrawal rate of over 20% and no RCT clearly described adequate precautions for the blinding of treatment allocation. We found no evidence comparing ziprasidone with other new antipsychotic drugs.

OPTION ZOTEPINE

One systematic review that compared zotepine with standard antipsychotic drugs found weak evidence that zotepine reduced a standard symptom severity score and had fewer adverse effects. This finding was not robust as removal of a single RCT altered the conclusion. We found no evidence comparing zotepine with other new antipsychotic drugs.

Benefits: We found one systematic review (search date 1999, 10 RCTs, 537 people).[28] **Versus standard antipsychotic drugs:** The systematic review included eight RCTs comparing zotepine (75–450 mg daily) versus a variety of standard antipsychotic drugs. Zotepine was more likely than standard antipsychotic drugs to bring about "clinically important improvement" as defined by a pre-stated cut off point on the brief psychiatric rating scale (356 people: 4 RCTs; RR 1.25, 95% CI 1.1 to 1.4; NNT 7, 95% CI 4 to 22).

Harms: The review found zotepine caused less akathisia (396 people: RR 0.7, 95% CI 0.6 to 0.9; NNT 8, 95% CI 5 to 34), dystonia (70 people: RR 0.5, 95% CI 0.2 to 0.9; NNT 4, 95% CI 2 to 56), and rigidity (164 people: RR 0.6, 95% CI 0.4 to 0.9; NNT 7, 95% CI 4 to 360) than standard antipsychotic drugs.[28]

Comment: All but one trial were of 12 weeks or less duration and all were conducted in Europe. Only one RCT favoured zotepine over standard antipsychotic drugs, and removal of this RCT from the analysis changed the result from a significant to a non-significant effect. Two RCTs found abnormal electrocardiogram results in people taking zotepine, but few additional details were given. We found too few trials to compare zotepine reliably with other new antipsychotics.

OPTION   CLOZAPINE

Two systematic reviews have found some evidence that clozapine may be more effective than standard antipsychotic drugs. However, clozapine is associated with potentially fatal blood dyscrasias. Three systematic reviews of RCTs found no strong evidence about the effectiveness or safety of clozapine compared with new antipsychotic drugs.

Benefits: We found four systematic reviews.[18,21,22,29] **Versus standard antipsychotics:** One systematic review (search date 1999, 31 RCTs, 2530 people, 73% men) compared clozapine versus standard antipsychotics, such as chlorpromazine and haloperidol. It found that clozapine was associated with greater clinical improvement both in the short term (4–10 wks, 14 RCTs, 1131 people: RR no important improvement 0.7, 95% CI 0.7 to 0.8; NNT 6, 95% CI 5 to 7) and the long term (heterogeneous data).[29] One additional systematic review (search date 1998, 12 RCTs) similarly found that clozapine improved symptoms compared with standard antipsychotics (WMD –0.68, 95% CI –0.82 to –0.55, indicating that 75% of people taking standard antipsychotics had worse composite symptom scores than those taking clozapine). However, the two included long term trials were heterogeneous and the short term benefit was not observed after controlling for the dose of standard drug (see benefits of amisulpride, p 134).[18] **Versus new antipsychotics:** We found one systematic review (search date 1999, 8 RCTs), which compared clozapine versus new antipsychotics, including olanzapine and risperidone,[21] and two systematic reviews, which included comparisons of clozapine versus risperidone (search date 1999, 5 RCTs;[22] search date 1998, 2 RCTs[18]). All three systematic reviews found no significant difference in efficacy, but the number of people studied was too small to rule out a clinically important difference.

Harms: **Versus standard antipsychotics:** Clozapine was more likely to cause hypersalivation (1419 people: RR 3.0, 95% CI 1.8 to 4.7; NNH 3), temperature increases (1147 people: RR 1.8, 95% CI 1.2 to 2.7; NNH 11), and sedation (1527 people: RR 1.2, 95% CI 1.1 to 1.4; NNH 10), but less likely to cause dry mouth (799 people: RR 0.4, 95% CI 0.3 to 0.6; NNT 6), and extrapyramidal adverse effects (1235 people: RR 0.7, 95% CI 0.5 to 0.9; NNT 6).[18] One systematic review found blood problems occurred more frequently with clozapine than with standard antipsychotics (1293 people: AR 3.6% v 1.9%; NNH 58, 95% CI 31 to 111).[29] In a large observational case series, leucopenia was reported in 3% of 99 502 people over 5 years. However, it found monitoring white cell (neutrophil) counts was associated with a lower than expected rate of cases of agranulocytosis (382 v 995; AR 0.38% v 1%) and deaths (12 v 149).[30] Dyscrasias were more common in younger people in a single RCT included in the first systematic review (21 people: RR 5.4, 95% CI 10 to 162; NNH 2.5).[29,31] One review found that, despite the requirement for regular blood tests, fewer people withdrew from treatment with clozapine in the long term (1513 people: RR 0.8, 95% CI 0.6 to 0.9; NNH 3).[29] However, another review found that long term drop out rate was only lower on fixed effects but not on random effects analyses. The difference in drop out rates did not persist after controlling for dose of haloperidol in an meta-regression analysis of all new antipsychotics considered together.[18] **Versus new antipsychotics:** Compared with new antipsychotic drugs (mainly risperidone), clozapine was less likely to cause extrapyramidal adverse effects (305 people: RR 0.3, 95% CI 0.1 to 0.6; NNT 6, 95% CI 4 to 9). Clozapine may also be less likely to cause dry mouth and more likely to cause fatigue, nausea, dizziness, hypersalivation, and hypersomnia, but these findings were from one or at most two trials.[21] Compared with new antipsychotics, people on clozapine tended to be more satisfied with their treatment, but also tended to withdraw from trials more easily.[21] Two reviews found no difference in rates of blood dyscrasias between clozapine and the new antipsychotics, but the number of people studied was too small (558) to rule out clinically important differences.[21,22]

Comment: Some of the benefits of clozapine were more apparent in the long term, depending on which drug was used for comparison in the trials.

QUESTION   **Which interventions reduce relapse rates?**

OPTION   **CONTINUED TREATMENT WITH ANTIPSYCHOTIC DRUGS**

Systematic reviews have found that continuing antipsychotic medication for at least 6 months after an acute episode significantly reduces relapse rates, and that some benefit of continuing treatment is apparent for up to 2 years. We found no evidence of a difference in relapse rates among standard antipsychotic drugs, but a systematic review has found that relapse rates are lower with clozapine.

Benefits: **Versus no treatment or placebo:** We found three systematic reviews.[6,8,32] All found evidence that continued treatment was beneficial for prevention of relapse. One review (search date not stated, 66 studies, 4365 people taking antipsychotic drugs, mean dose 630 mg chlorpromazine equivalents daily, mean follow up of 6.3 months) included 29 controlled trials with a mean follow up of 9.7 months.[32] It found significantly lower relapse in 1224 people maintained on treatment compared with 1224 withdrawn from treatment (16.2% v 51.5%; ARR 35%, 95% CI 33% to 38%; NNT 3,

Schizophrenia

95% CI 2.6 to 3.1). Over time, the relapse rate in people maintained on antipsychotic treatment approached that in those withdrawn from treatment, but was still lower in those on treatment at 2 years (ARR 22%; NNT 5). The second review (search date 1997) found that relapse rates over 6–24 months were significantly lower on chlorpromazine than placebo (3 heterogeneous RCTs; RR 0.7, 95% CI 0.5 to 0.9; NNT 3, 95% CI 2.5 to 4).[6] One subsequent systematic review (search date 1998, 20 RCTs) comparing haloperidol with placebo included two RCTs (70 people currently in remission; duration 1 year). Haloperidol was more effective than placebo for preventing relapse (ARR 33%, 95% CI 16% to 50%; NNT 4, 95% CI 2 to 7).[8] **Choice of drug:** We found 10 systematic reviews, which found that the choice of drug or preparation did not seem to affect relapse rates. The first systematic review (search date 1995) identified six RCTs comparing oral with depot fluphenazine (see table 1, p 151).[33] A second systematic review (search date 1998) identified seven RCTs comparing haloperidol decanoate with other depot antipsychotics.[10] A third systematic review (search date 1998) identified eight RCTs comparing flupentixol (flupenthixol) decanoate with other depot antipsychotics.[34] A fourth systematic review (search date 1998, 14 RCTs) identified seven RCTs (417 people) comparing pipotiazine palmitate with other depots, and one RCT (124 people) comparing pipotiazine palmitate with oral antipsychotics.[11] A fifth systematic review (search date 1998) identified one RCT comparing fluspirilene decanoate with oral chlorpromazine, and three RCTs comparing fluspirilene decanoate with other depot preparations.[35] A sixth systematic review (search date 1998) found one RCT comparing perphenazine enanthate with clopenthixol decanoate.[36] The reviews comparing pimozide and olanzapine versus typical antipsychotic drugs also found no significant difference in relapse rates.[14,19] The number of people studied was too small to rule out clinically important differences. One systematic review (search date 1998) comparing clozapine with standard antipsychotic drugs found that relapse rates up to 12 weeks were significantly lower with clozapine (19 RCTs; RR 0.6, 95% CI 0.5 to 0.8; NNT 20).[29] Another systematic review (search date 1998) found that significantly fewer people taking depot zuclopenthixol decanoate relapsed over 12 weeks to 1 year compared with people taking other depot preparations (3 RCTs, 296 people: RR 0.7, 95% CI 0.6 to 1.0; NNT 9, 95% CI 5 to 53).[37]

Harms: Mild transient nausea, malaise, sweating, vomiting, insomnia, and dyskinesia were reported in an unspecified number of people after sudden drug cessation, but were usually acceptable with gradual dose reduction.[38] Annual incidence of tardive dyskinesia was 5%.[37]

Comment: In the systematic review of continued treatment versus withdrawal of treatment, meta-analysis of the 29 controlled trials gave similar results to those obtained when all 66 studies were included (ARR 37%, NNT 3).[37] The review was weakened because all RCT results were used rather than weighted comparisons, no length of time was given since the last acute episode, and no distinction was made between people experiencing a first episode and those with chronic illness.[37] Some clinicians use depot antipsychotic medication in selected people to ensure adherence to medication. We found no evidence from RCTs to support this practice.

| OPTION | FAMILY INTERVENTIONS |

One systematic review has found that family intervention significantly reduces relapse rates compared with usual care.

Benefits: We found one systematic review (search date 1998, 13 RCTs),[39] and one additional RCT comparing family interventions with usual care.[40] Family interventions consisted mainly of education about the illness and training in problem solving over at least six weekly sessions. Three of the trials included substantial proportions of people experiencing their first episode. Family interventions significantly reduced relapse rates at 12 and 24 months. At 12 months, the risk of relapse was reduced (6 RCTs, 516 people: RR 0.7, 95% CI 0.5 to 1.0), such that seven families would have to be treated to avoid one additional relapse (and likely hospitalisation) in the family member with schizophrenia (NNT 7, 95% CI 4 to 14).[41] We found one potentially relevant additional RCT of family interventions compared with psychoeducation, which is being assessed.[42]

Harms: No harms were reported, although illness education could possibly have adverse consequences on morale and outlook.[41]

Comment: These results are likely to overestimate treatment effect because of the difficulty of blinding people and investigators and the likelihood of publication bias.[39] The trend over time is for results to tend to the null. The mechanism for the effects of family intervention remains unclear. It is thought to work by reducing "expressed emotion" (hostility and criticism) in relatives of people with schizophrenia. The time consuming nature of this intervention, which must normally take place at evenings or weekends, can limit its availability. It cannot be applied to people who have little contact with home based carers.

| OPTION | SOCIAL SKILLS TRAINING |

Limited evidence from RCTs suggests that social skills training may reduce relapse rates.

Benefits: We found one non-systematic review and meta-analysis of 27 RCTs (search date not stated) comparing social skills training with usual care.[43] The trials were mainly in men admitted to hospital, not all of whom had schizophrenia, using different techniques that generally included instruction in social interaction. Four studies provided quantitative information, of which three defined relapse as rehospitalisation. Social skills training significantly reduced relapse rates (WMD 0.47). However, sensitivity analysis indicated that five null results (in studies not identified by a search) would render the difference non-significant. One systematic review (search date 1988) identified 73 RCTs in people with a variety of psychiatric disorders and found similar results, but suggested that motivation was an important predictor of benefit from treatment.[44]

Harms: None reported.

Comment: Many of the trials simultaneously compared the effects of other interventions (medication, education), so the effects of individual interventions are difficult to assess. Overall, it remains uncertain whether people at different stages of illness and function require different approaches. Selected people may benefit even from interventions of short duration.

OPTION | **COGNITIVE BEHAVIOURAL THERAPY**

Limited evidence from RCTs suggests that cognitive behavioural therapy may reduce relapse rates.

Benefits: We found one systematic review (search date 1998, 4 small RCTs) comparing cognitive behavioural therapy plus standard care with standard care alone.[45] All trials incorporated the challenging of key beliefs, problem solving, and enhancement of coping. Relapse rates were significantly reduced in the short, medium, and long term. In the long term (up to 18 months), cognitive behavioural therapy plus standard care reduced the risk of relapse (3 RCTs, 183 people: RR 0.7, 95% CI 0.5 to 0.9; NNT 6, 95% CI 3 to 30).

Harms: None reported.

Comment: None of the three trials contributing long term results was blinded, and each concentrated on different clinical issues — symptoms, adherence to treatment, or general rehabilitation. The fourth trial blinded outcome raters and included an additional supportive psychotherapy control group. It found non-significantly lower relapse rates with cognitive behavioural therapy (1 RCT, 59 people: RR 0.6, 95% CI 0.2 to 2.1).

OPTION | **PSYCHOEDUCATIONAL INTERVENTIONS**

One systematic review has found that psychoeducation is effective for preventing relapse.

Benefits: **Versus usual treatment:** We found one systematic review (search date 1999, 10 RCTs, 1128 people, 53% male).[46] The systematic review included one RCT of a brief individual intervention (10 sessions or less), but no standard length individual psychoeducational interventions (11 sessions or more). It included six RCTs of brief group psychoeducational interventions and four of standard length. Standard length interventions were significantly more effective than treatment as usual in preventing relapse during 9–18 months (6 RCTs, 720 people: RR 0.80, 95% CI 0.70 to 0.92; NNT 6, 95% CI 3 to 83). Brief group psychoeducational interventions were also more effective than treatment as usual in preventing relapse or re admission by 1 year (RR 0.85, 95% CI 0.74 to 0.98; NNT 12 CI 6 to 83). When all trials were pooled, relapse rates at 9–18 months' follow up were significantly lower in the psychoeducation group than in the control intervention group (6 RCTs; RR 0.80, 95% CI 0.70 to 0.92; NNT 9, 95% CI 6 to 22).

Harms: None reported.

Comment: The systematic review found few good RCTs. There was significant heterogeneity of both interventions and outcomes.

Which interventions are effective in people resistant to standard treatment?

One systematic review has found that clozapine benefits people who are resistant to standard treatment.

Benefits: **Clozapine:** We found one systematic review (search date 1999, 6 RCTs) comparing clozapine versus standard antipsychotic drugs in people who were resistant to standard treatment.[29] Clozapine achieved improvement both in the short term (6–12 wks, 4 RCTs, 370 people: RR for no improvement compared with standard antipsychotic drugs 0.7, 95% CI 0.6 to 0.8; NNT 5), and in the longer term (12–24 months: 2 RCTs, 648 people: RR 0.8, 95% CI 0.6 to 1.0). There was no difference in relapse rates in the short term. **Other interventions:** We found no good evidence on the effects of other interventions in people resistant to standard treatment.

Harms: See harms of clozapine, p 140.

Comment: Trials are under way to clarify the mode of action of cognitive behavioural therapy and establish its effects in people who are resistant to standard treatments.

Which interventions improve adherence to antipsychotic medication?

COMPLIANCE THERAPY

We found limited evidence from three RCTs that compliance therapy may increase adherence with antipsychotic medication.

Benefits: We found no systematic review. We found one RCT of compliance therapy (see glossary, p 147) versus supportive counselling, which included 47 people with acute psychoses, although the majority fulfilled criteria for schizophrenia or had been admitted with the first episode of a psychotic illness.[41,47] People treated with compliance therapy were significantly more likely to attain at least passive acceptance of antipsychotic medication versus people who received non-specific counselling, both immediately after the intervention (OR 6.3, 95% CI 1.6 to 24.6) and at 6 months' follow up (OR 5.2, 95% CI 1.5 to 18.3). At 18 months (for an extended sample of 74 people), a significant improvement on a seven point scale of medication adherence was found for people treated with compliance therapy (mean difference 1.4, 95% CI 0.9 to 1.6).

Harms: None reported.

Comment: Other trials have examined the potential benefits of compliance therapy, but either did not employ a standardised measure of adherence or adherence was not rated in a blind fashion. The RCT above requires independent replication. About a third of each group did not complete the trials, and missing data are estimated from the mean scores in each group. Calculation of numbers needed to treat was not possible because of missing data.

| OPTION | FAMILY THERAPY |

One systematic review has found that family therapy is unlikely to improve adherence with antipsychotic medication.

Benefits: We found one systematic review (search date 1998) comparing family therapy with usual care.[39] Family interventions consisted mainly of education about the illness and training in problem solving over at least six weekly sessions. "Poor compliance with medication" (5 RCTs, 257 people, 9 months' to 2 years' duration) and "poor compliance with treatment protocol" (12 RCTs, 745 people) were not altered by family therapy compared with usual care (OR for poor compliance with medication: family therapy v control 0.63, 95% CI 0.38 to 1.03; OR for poor compliance with treatment protocol: family therapy v control 1.10, 95% CI 0.72 to 1.66).

Harms: No harms were reported, although illness education could possibly have adverse consequences on morale and outlook.[39]

Comment: None.

| OPTION | PSYCHOEDUCATIONAL THERAPY |

One systematic review found limited evidence that psychoeducation improved adherence with antipsychotic medication.

Benefits: **Versus usual treatment:** We found one systematic review (search date 1999, 10 RCTs, 1128 people, 53% male).[46] The systematic review considered individual and group psychoeducation of either standard length (11 sessions or more) or brief interventional types (10 sessions or less). One trial (67 people with DSM-III-R schizophrenia) measured the effect of individual psychoeducation on compliance. It found no significant differences between the brief individual psychoeducation and treatment as usual on the compliance subscale of the schedule for assessment of insight. Two RCTs compared brief group psychoeducational interventions versus control group. Both suggest psychoeducation to be more effective than the comparison treatment. The first RCT (236 people) found a significant advantage group of psychoeducational intervention versus usual treatment on a continuous scale of medication concordance (WMD −0.4, 95% CI −0.6 to −0.2). The second RCT (46 people) of a brief psychoeducational intervention versus usual treatment reported compliance episodes at 1 year follow up. Skewed data suggested an advantage of psychoeducational interventions (treatment group: 24 people, mean number of non-compliant episodes at 1 year 0.38; control group: 22 people, mean 1.14). One trial (82 people, 18 months' duration) compared standard length group interventions versus treatment as usual and found no significant differences in compliance. **Versus behavioural therapy:** We found two RCTs.[48,49] One RCT (36 men) compared behavioural therapy versus psychoeducation versus usual treatment.[48] The behavioural training method comprised being told the importance of complying with antipsychotic medication and instructions on how to take medication. Each participant was given a self monitoring spiral calendar, which featured a dated slip of paper for each dose of antipsychotic. Adherence was estimated by pill counts. After 3 months, fewer people had high pill adherence after psychoeducation compared with behaviour therapy (3/11 v 8/11 had pill adherence scores of 80% measured by pill counts). The second RCT (39 people) compared a behavioural intervention given individually, a behavioural intervention involving the person with schizophrenia and their family, and a psychoeducational intervention.[49] The behavioural intervention consisted of specific written guidelines, and oral instructions, given to people to use a pill box consisting of 28 compartments for every medication occasion during a week. The behavioural intervention, when given to the individual and their family, also consisted of instructions for the family member to compliment the person with schizophrenia for taking their prescribed medication. The primary outcome measure was pill count at 2 months. Medication adherence was more likely with behavioural interventions than with psychoeducation (> 90% adherence at 2 months, 25/26 [96%] with behavioural methods v 6/13 [46%] with psychoeducation; ARR 0.5; RR 2.1; NNT 2 95% CI 2 to 5).

Harms: None reported.

Comment: There are few RCTs of psychoeducational interventions and most do not measure medication adherence. Each psychoeducational intervention varied in the protocol used and few employed the same outcome ratings.

OPTION   BEHAVIOURAL THERAPY

One RCT found that behavioural interventions improved adherence to antipsychotic medication compared with usual treatment. One RCT found that behavioural interventions improved adherence compared with psychoeducational therapy.

Benefits: We found no systematic review. **Versus usual treatment:** We found one RCT (36 men).[48] The behavioural training method comprised being told the importance of complying with antipsychotic medication and instructions on how to take medication. Each participant was given a self monitoring spiral calendar, which featured a dated slip of paper for each dose of antipsychotic. Adherence was estimated by pill counts. After 3 months fewer people had high pill adherence after usual treatment compared with behaviour therapy (figures not provided). **Versus psychoeducational therapy:** See benefits of psychoeducational therapy, p 146.

Harms: None reported.

Comment: See above.

GLOSSARY

Compliance therapy A treatment based on cognitive behavioural therapy and motivational interviewing techniques with a view to improving concordance to medication.

Schizophrenia

Mental health

Negative symptoms This generally refers to qualities abnormal by their absence (e.g. loss of drive, motivation, and self care).

Positive symptoms This refers to symptoms that characterise the onset or relapse of schizophrenia, usually hallucinations and delusions, but sometimes including thought disorder.

REFERENCES

1. Andreasen NC. Symptoms, signs and diagnosis of schizophrenia. *Lancet* 1995;346:477–481.
2. Cannon M, Jones P. Neuroepidemiology: schizophrenia. *J Neurol Neurosurg Psychiatry* 1996;61:604–613.
3. Jablensky A, Sartorius N, Ernberg G, et al. Schizophrenia: manifestations, incidence and course in different cultures. A World Health Organisation ten-country study. *Psychol Med* 1992;monograph supplement 20:1–97.
4. Hegarty JD, Baldessarini RJ, Tohen M, Waternaux C, Oepen G. One hundred years of schizophrenia: a meta-analysis of the outcome literature. *Am J Psychiatry* 1994;151:1409–1416.
5. Johnstone EC. Schizophrenia: problems in clinical practice. *Lancet* 1993; 341:536–538.
6. Thornley B, Adams C. Content and quality of 2000 controlled trials in schizophrenia over 50 years. *BMJ* 1998;317:1181–1184. Search date 1997; primary sources hand searching of conference proceedings, Biological Abstracts, Cinahl, The Cochrane Library (Issue 3, 1997), Embase, Lilacs, Psychlit, Pstndex, Medline, and Sociofile.
7. Thornley B, Adams CE, Awad G. Chlorpromazine versus placebo for those with schizophrenia. In: The Cochrane Library, Issue 3, 2001. Oxford: Update Software. Search date 1999; primary sources Biological Abstracts, Embase, Medline, Psychlit, SciSearch, Cochrane Library, Cochrane Schizophrenia Group's Register, hand searches of reference lists, and personal contact with pharmaceutical companies and authors of trials.
8. Joy CB, Adams CE, Lawrie SM. Haloperidol versus placebo for schizophrenia. In: The Cochrane Library, Issue 3, 2001. Oxford: Update Software. Search date 1998; primary sources Biological Abstracts, Cinahl, The Cochrane Schizophrenia Group's Register, Embase, Medline, Psychlit, SciSearch, hand searches of references, and contact with authors of trials and pharmaceutical companies.
9. Sultana A, Reilly J, Fenton M. Thioridazine for schizophrenia. In: The Cochrane Library, Issue 3, 2001. Oxford: Update Software. Search date 1999; primary sources Biological Abstracts, Cinahl, The Cochrane Library, The Cochrane Schizophrenia Group's Register, Embase, Psychlit, Sociofile, reference lists, pharmaceutical companies, and authors of trials.
10. Quraishi S, David A. Depot haloperidol decanoate for schizophrenia. In: The Cochrane Library, Issue 3, 2001. Oxford: Update Software. Search date 1998; primary sources Biological Abstracts, Embase, Medline, Psychlit, SciSearch, The Cochrane Library, reference lists, authors of studies, and pharmaceutical companies.
11. Quraishi S, David A. Depot pipothiazine palmitate and undeclynate for schizophrenia. In: The Cochrane Library, Issue 3, 2001. Oxford: Update Software. Search date 1998; primary sources Biological Abstracts, Cochrane Library, Cochrane Schizophrenia Group's Register, Embase, Medline, Psychlit, hand searches of reference lists, and personal communication with pharmaceutical companies.
12. Fenton M, Murphy B, Wood J, Bagnell AM, Schou P, Leitner M. Loxapine for schizophrenia. In: The

Cochrane Library, Issue 3, 2001. Oxford: Update Software. Search date 1999; primary sources Biological Abstracts, The Cochrane Library, The Cochrane Schizophrenia Group's Register, Embase, Lilacs, Psyndex, Psychlit, and hand searches of reference lists.
13. Bagnall AM, Fenton M, Lewis R, Leitner ML, Kleijnen J. Molindone for schizophrenia and severe mental illness. In: The Cochrane Library, Issue 3, 2001. Oxford: Update Software. Search date 1999; primary sources Biological Abstracts, The Cochrane Library, The Cochrane Schizophrenia Group's Register, Cinahl, Embase, Psychlit, pharmaceutical databases, hand searches of reference lists, and personal contact with authors of trials.
14. Sultana A, McMonagle T. Pimozide for schizophrenia or related psychoses. In: The Cochrane Library, Issue 3, 2001. Oxford: Update Software. Search date 1999; primary sources Biological Abstracts, The Cochrane Schizophrenia Group's Register, Embase, Janssen-Cilag UK's register of studies, Medline, hand searches of reference lists, and personal contact with pharmaceutical companies.
15. Joy CB, Mumby-Croft R, Joy LA. Polyunsaturated fatty acid (fish or evening primrose oil) for schizophrenia. In: The Cochrane Library, Issue 3, 2001. Oxford: Update Software. Search date 2000; primary sources Biological Abstracts, Cinahl, The Cochrane Library, The Cochrane Schizophrenia Group's Register, Embase, Psychlit, hand searches of reference lists and personal contact with the authors.
16. Soares BGO, Fenton M, Chue P. Sulpiride for schizophrenia. In: The Cochrane Library, Issue 3, 2001. Oxford: Update Software. Search date 1998; primary sources Biological Abstracts, Cinahl, Cochrane Schizophrenia Group's Register, The Cochrane Library, Embase, Medline, Psychlit, Sigle, and Sociofile.
17. Harnryd C, et al. Clinical evaluation of sulpiride in schizophrenic patients — a double-blind comparison with chlorpromazine. *Acta Psych Scand.* 1984;311:7–30.
18. Geddes J, Freemantle N, Harrison P, Bebbington P, for the National Schizophrenia Development Group. Atypical antipsychotics in the treatment of schizophrenia: systematic review and meta-regression analysis. *BMJ* 2000;321:1371–1377. Search date 1998; primary sources Medline, Embase, Psychlit, and Cochrane Controlled Trials Register.
19. Duggan L, Fenton M, Dardennes RM, El-Dosoky A, Indran S. Olanzapine for schizophrenia. In: The Cochrane Library, Issue 3, 2001. Oxford: Update Software. Search date 1999; primary sources Biological Abstracts, Embase, Medline, Psychlit, Cochrane Library, hand searches of reference lists and conference abstracts, and personal communication with authors of trials and pharmaceutical companies.
20. Leucht S, Pitschel-Walx G, Abraham D, Kissling W. Efficacy and extrapyramidal side-effects of the new antipsychotics olanzapine, quetiapine, risperidone and sertindole compared to conventional antipsychotics and placebo. A meta-analysis of

randomised controlled trials. *Schizophr Res* 1999; 35:51–68. Search date 1999; primary sources Medline, Current Contents, hand searches of reference lists, and personal communication with pharmaceutical companies.

21. Tuunainen A, Gilbody SM. Newer atypical antipsychotic medication versus clozapine for schizophrenia. In: The Cochrane Library, Issue 3, 2001. Oxford: Update Software. Search date 1998; primary sources Biological Abstracts, Cochrane Schizophrenia Group's Register, Cochrane Library, Embase, Lilacs, Medline, Psychlit, hand searches of reference lists, and personal contact with authors of trials and pharmaceutical companies.

22. Gilbody SM, Bagnall AM, Duggan L, Tuunainen A. Risperidone versus other atypical antipsychotic medication for schizophrenia. In: The Cochrane Library, Issue 3, 2001. Oxford: Update Software. Search date 1999; primary sources Biological Abstracts, Cochrane Library, Cochrane Schizophrenia Group's Register, Embase, Medline, Lilacs, Psyindex, Psychlit, pharmaceutical databases on the Dialog Corporation Datastar and Dialog services, hand search of reference lists, and contact with pharmaceutical companies and authors of trials.

23. Conley RR, Mahmoud R. A randomized double-blind study of risperidone and olanzapine in the treatment of schizophrenia or schizoaffective disorder. *Am J Psychiatry* 2001;158:765–774.

24. Srisurapanont M, Disayavanish C, Taimkaew K. Quetiapine for schizophrenia. In: The Cochrane Library, Issue 3, 2001. Oxford: Update Software. Search date 2000; primary sources Biological Abstracts, Embase, Medline, Psychlit, The Cochrane Library, Cinahl, Sigle, Sociofile, hand searches of journals, and personal communication with authors of studies and pharmaceutical companies.

25. Kennedy E, Song F, Hunter R, Clarke Q, Gilbody S. Risperidone versus typical antipsychotic medication for schizophrenia. In: The Cochrane Library, Issue 3, 2001. Oxford: Update Software. Search date 1997; primary sources Biological Abstracts, The Cochrane Trials Register, Embase, Medline, Psychlit, hand searches of reference lists, and personal communication with pharmaceutical companies.

26. Lopez Ibor JJ, Ayuso JL, Gutierrez M, et al. Risperidone in the treatment of chronic schizophrenia: multicenter study comparative to haloperidol. *Actas Luso Esp Neurol Psiquiatr Cienc Afines* 1996;24:165–172.

27. Bagnall AM, Lewis RA, Leitner ML, Kleijnen J. Ziprasidone for schizophrenia and severe mental illness. In: The Cochrane Library, Issue 3, 2001. Oxford: Update Software. Search date 1999; primary sources Biological Abstracts, The Cochrane Library, The Cochrane Schizophrenia Group's Register, Embase, Lilacs, Psyndex, Psychlit, pharmaceutical databases, hand searches of reference lists, and personal contact with authors of trials.

28. Fenton M, Morris F, De Silva P, et al. Zotepine for schizophrenia. In: The Cochrane Library, Issue 3, 2001. Oxford: Update Software. Search date 1999; primary sources Biological Abstracts, The Cochrane Library, The Cochrane Schizophrenia Group's Register, Embase, Dialog Corporation Datastar service, Medline, Psychlit, hand searches of reference lists, and personal contact with authors of trials and pharmaceutical companies.

29. Wahlbeck K, Cheine M, Essali MA. Clozapine versus typical neuroleptic medication for schizophrenia. In: The Cochrane Library, Issue 3, 2001. Oxford: Update Software. Search date 1999; primary sources Biological Abstracts, Cochrane Schizophrenia Group's Register, Cochrane Library, Embase, Lilacs, Medline, Psychlit, SciSearch Science Citation Index, hand searches of reference lists, and personal communication with pharmaceutical companies.

30. Honigfeld G, Arellano F, Sethi J, Bianchini A, Schein J. Reducing clozapine-related morbidity and mortality: five years experience of the clozaril national registry. *J Clin Psychiatry* 1998;59(suppl 3):3–7.

31. Kumra S, Frazier JA, Jacobsen LK, et al. Childhood-onset schizophrenia. A double-blind clozapine-haloperidol comparison. *Arch Gen Psychiatry* 1996;53:1090–1097.

32. Gilbert PL, Harris MJ, McAdams LA, Jeste DV. Neuroleptic withdrawal in schizophrenic people: a review of the literature. *Arch Gen Psychiatry* 1995; 52:173–188. Search date not stated; primary source Medline.

33. Adams CE, Eisenbruch M. Depot fluphenazine versus oral fluphenazine for those with schizophrenia. In: The Cochrane Library, Issue 3, 2001. Oxford: Update Software. Search date 1995; primary sources Biological Abstracts, The Cochrane Library, Cochrane Schizophrenia Group's Register, Embase, Medline, Psychlit, Science Citation Index, hand searches of reference lists, and personal communication with pharmaceutical companies.

34. Quraishi S, David A. Depot flupenthixol decanoate for schizophrenia or similar psychotic disorders. In: The Cochrane Library, Issue 3, 2001. Oxford: Update Software. Search date 1998; primary sources Biological Abstracts, The Cochrane Library, Cochrane Schizophrenia Group's Register, Embase, Medline, Psychlit, SciSearch, references, and personal communication with authors of trials and pharmaceutical companies.

35. Quraishi S, David A. Depot fluspirilene for schizophrenia. In: The Cochrane Library, Issue 3, 2001. Oxford: Update Software. Search date 1998; primary sources Biological Abstracts, The Cochrane Library, The Cochrane Schizophrenia Group's Register, Embase, Medline, Psychlit, and hand searches of reference lists.

36. Quraishi S, David A. Depot perphenazine decanoate and enanthate for schizophrenia. In: The Cochrane Library, Issue 3, 2001. Oxford: Update Software. Search date 1998; primary sources Biological Abstracts, The Cochrane Library, The Cochrane Schizophrenia Group's Register, Embase, Medline, Psychlit, hand searches of reference lists, and personal communication with pharmaceutical companies.

37. Coutinho E, Fenton M, Quraishi S. Zuclopenthixol decanoate for schizophrenia and other serious mental illnesses. In: The Cochrane Library, Issue 3, 2001. Oxford: Update Software. Search date 1998; primary sources Biological Abstracts, Cinhal, The Cochrane Library, The Cochrane Schizophrenia Group's Register, Embase, Medline, and Psychlit. References of all eligible studies were searched for further trials. The manufacturer of zuclopenthixol was contacted.

38. Jeste D, Gilbert P, McAdams L, Harris M. Considering neuroleptic maintenance and taper on a continuum: need for an individual rather than dogmatic approach. *Arch Gen Psychiatry* 1995; 52:209–212.

39. Pharoah FM, Mari JJ, Streiner D. Family intervention for schizophrenia. In: The Cochrane Library, Issue 3, 2001. Oxford: Update Software. Search date 1998; primary sources Medline, Embase, The Cochrane Library, Cochrane Schizophrenia Group's Register, and reference lists of articles.

40. McFarlane WR, Lukens E, Link B, et al. Multiple-family groups and psychoeducation in the treatment of schizophrenia. *Arch Gen Psychiatry* 1995;52:679–687.

41. Kemp R, Kirov G, Everitt B, Hayward P, David A. Randomised controlled trial of compliance therapy. 18-month follow-up. *Br J Psychiatry* 1998;172: 413–419.

42. Strang JS, Falloon IRH, Moss HB, Razani J, Boyd JL. Drug treatment and family intervention during the aftercare treatment of schizophrenics. *Psychopharmacology Bull* 1981;17:87–88.

43. Benton MK, Schroeder HE. Social skills training with schizophrenics: a meta-analytic evaluation. *J Consult Clin Psychol* 1990;58:741–747. Search date not stated; primary sources computerised databases and manual search but sources not specified.

44. Corrigan PW. Social skills training in adult psychiatric populations: a meta-analysis. *J Behav Ther Exp Psychiatry* 1991;22:203–210. Search date 1988; primary source Psychological Abstracts.

45. Jones C, Cormac I, Mota J, Campbell C. Cognitive behavioural therapy for schizophrenia. In: The Cochrane Library, Issue 3, 2001. Oxford: Update Software. Search date 1998; primary sources Biological Abstracts, Cochrane Schizophrenia Group's Register, Cinahl, The Cochrane Library, Medline, Embase, Psychlit, Sigle, Sociofile, reference lists of articles, and personal communication with authors of trials.

46. Pekkala E, Merinder L. Psychoeducation for schizophrenia. In: The Cochrane Library, Issue 3, 2001. Oxford: Update Software. Search date 1999; primary sources Cinahl, The Cochrane Library, Cochrane Schizophrenia Group's Register, Embase, Medline, Psychlit, Sociofile, hand searched reference lists, and personal contact with authors.

47. Kemp R, Hayward P, Applewhaite G, Everitt B, David A. Compliance therapy in psychotic people: randomised controlled trial. *BMJ* 1996;312: 345–349.

48. Boczkowski JA, Zeichner A, DeSanto N. Neuroleptic compliance among chronic schizophrenic outpeople: an intervention outcome report. *J Consult Clin Psychol* 1985;53:666–671.

49. Azrin NH, Teichner G. Evaluation of an instructional program for improving medication compliance for chronically mentally ill outpatients. *Behaviour Res Ther* 1998;36:849–861.

Stephen Lawrie

Senior Clinical Research Fellow and
Honorary Consultant Psychiatrist

Andrew McIntosh

Lecturer in Psychiatry
Department of Psychiatry
University of Edinburgh
Edinburgh
UK

Competing interests: SML has been paid for speaking about critical appraisal by employees of the manufacturers of olanzapine, quetiapine, risperidone, and ziprasidone, and has been paid to speak about the management of schizophrenia by employees of the manufacturers of amisulpiride, olanzapine, risperidone, and clozapine. AM, none declared.

TABLE 1 Continued treatment with antipsychotic drugs: choice of drugs (see text, p 142).

Review	Search Date	Number of RCTs	Comparisons	Main Conclusion
33	1995	6	Oral v depot fluphenazine	No significant difference
10	1998	7	Haloperidol decanoate v other depots	No significant difference
34	1999	8	Flupenthixol decanoate v other depots	No significant difference
11	1999	7	Pipothiazine palmitate v other depots	No significant difference
11	1999	2	Pipothiazine palmitate v oral antipsychotics	No significant difference
35	1999	1	Fluspirilene decanoate v oral chlorpromazine	No significant difference
35	1999	3	Fluspirilene decanoate v other depots	No significant difference
36	1999	1	Perphenazine enanthate v clopenthixol decanoate	No significant difference
14	2000	11	Pimozide v standard antipsychotics	No significant difference
19	1999	1	Olanzapine v standard antipsychotics	No significant difference
37	1998	3	Zuclopenthixol decanoate v other depots	People taking zuclopenthixol had lower relapse rates over 12 weeks to 1 year
29	1999	19	Clozapine v standard antipsychotics	Relapse rates up to 12 weeks were lower with clozapine

Note

When looking up a class of drug, the reader is advised to also look up specific examples of that class of drug where additional entries may be found. The reverse situation also applies.

vs olanzapine 135–6
Cognitive behavioural therapy 29, 72, 118, 125
  adverse effects 25, 124
  bulimia nervosa 21, 23–5, 32
  chronic fatigue syndrome 33, 41–3
  depression 82
    children/adolescents 67, 70, 71
    post-traumatic stress disorder and 120, 121–2, 123
  pure self help cognitive behavioural therapy 30
  schizophrenia 128, 144
Cognitive orientation therapy 29
Cognitive therapy 18, 85, 110, 125
  anorexia nervosa 3
  depression 74, 82, 85, 89
    with drug treatment 83
  generalised anxiety disorder 90, 92–3
    vs relaxation therapy 92–3
  obsessive compulsive disorder 103, 108–9
    combination therapy 109
    vs behavioural therapy 108–9
Compliance therapy 147
  schizophrenia 128, 145
Compulsions 104
  see also Obsessive compulsive disorder
Conduct disorder 18
Conners Teacher Rating Scale 13, 15, 18
Continuation treatment 85
Corticosteroids, chronic fatigue syndrome treatment 33, 36–7
Counselling
  depression therapy 75, 82
  non-directive counselling 75, 82, 85, 89
  post-traumatic stress disorder and 120, 122
Cyproheptadine, anorexia nervosa treatment 1, 6
Debriefing 125
  adverse effects 121
  post-traumatic stress disorder prevention 120, 121–2
Dementia 46–61
  see also Alzheimer's disease
  aetiology/risk factors 48
  definition 47
  incidence/prevalence 48
  Lewy body dementia 47–8
  outcome measures 46
  prognosis 48
  treatment effects on behavioural and psychological symptoms 58–61
    antidepressants 60–1
    antiepileptics 60
    antipsychotics 58–60
    behaviour management 61
  treatment effects on cognition 47, 49–58
    donepezil 47, 49–50, 65
    galantamine 47, 51, 65
    ginkgo biloba 47, 56–7
    lecithin 47, 53
    music therapy 47, 57–8

nicotine 47, 53
NSAIDs 47, 53–4
physostigmine 47, 52–3
reality orientation 47, 57
reminiscence therapy 47, 57
rivastigmine 47, 50–1, 65
selegiline 47, 55–6
tacrine 47, 51–2
vascular dementia 47
Depression 18, 74–85
  aetiology/risk factors 68, 75
  antidepressant treatment 74, 75, 76–9
    continuation/maintenance treatment 75, 84–5
    in children/adolescents 67, 68–70
    with benzodiazepines 78
  befriending therapy 75, 84
  bibliotherapy 75, 84
  care pathways 79–80
  cognitive therapy 74, 82, 90
    in children/adolescents 67, 70, 71
    with drug treatment 83
  definition 68, 75
  electroconvulsive therapy 74, 81–2
    in children/adolescents 67, 70
  exercise and 75, 83
  family therapy 67, 71
  group therapy 67, 71
  in children and adolescents 67–71
  incidence/prevalence 75
    in children/adolescents 68
  interpersonal therapy 74, 82, 90
    in children/adolescents 67, 70–1
    with drug treatment 83
  non-directive counselling 75, 82, 90
  outcomes 76, 85
  problem solving therapy 74, 81, 90
  prognosis 68, 75
  psychological treatments 82–3, 90
    in children/adolescents 70–1
    with drug treatment 83
  St John's wort benefits 74, 80–1
    in children/adolescents 67, 70
  social skills training 71
Desipramine
  bulimia nervosa treatment 26–7
  obsessive compulsive disorder treatment 106
Dexamfetamine
  adverse effects 14, 15
  attention deficit hyperactivity disorder treatment 11, 15
  vs methylphenidate 13
Dialectical behaviour therapy 29
Diazepam, generalised anxiety disorder treatment 98
Diclofenac, Alzheimer's disease treatment 54
Dietary advice 8
Dietary intervention
  anorexia nervosa 1, 3–4
  chronic fatigue syndrome 33, 39–40
  schizophrenia 133
Donepezil
  adverse effects 49–50, 66

The number needed to treat: adjusting for baseline risk

Adapted with permission from Chatellier et al, 1996[1]

BACKGROUND

The number needed to treat (NNT) to avoid a single additional adverse outcome is a meaningful way of expressing the benefit of an active treatment over a control. It can be used both to summarise the results of a therapeutic trial or series of trials and to help medical decision making about an individual patient.

If the absolute risk of adverse outcomes in a therapeutic trial is ARC in the control group and ART in the treatment group, then the absolute risk reduction (ARR) is defined as (ARC − ART). The NNT is defined as the inverse of the ARR:

$$NNT = 1/(ARC - ART)$$

Since the Relative Risk Reduction (RRR) is defined as (ARC − ART)/ARC, it follows that NNT, RRR and ARC are related by their definitions in the following way:

$$NNT \times RRR \times ARC = 1$$

This relationship can be used to estimate the likely benefits of a treatment in populations with different levels of baseline risk (that is different levels of ARC). This allows extrapolation of the results of a trial or meta-analysis to people with different baseline risks. Ideally, there should be experimental evidence of the RRR in each population. However in many trials, subgroup analyses show that the RRR is approximately constant in groups of patients with different characteristics. Cook and Sackett therefore proposed that decisions about individual patients could be made by using the NNT calculated from the RRR measured in trials and the baseline risk in the absence of treatment estimated for the individual patient.[2]

The method may not apply to periods of time different to that studied in the original trials.

USING THE NOMOGRAM

The nomogram shown on the next page allows the NNT to be found directly without any calculation: a straight line should be drawn from the point corresponding to the estimated absolute risk for the patient on the left hand scale to the point corresponding to the relative risk reduction stated in a trial or meta-analysis on the central scale. The intercept of this line with the right hand scale gives the NNT. By taking the upper and lower limits of the confidence interval of the RRR, the upper and lower limits of the NNT can be estimated.

REFERENCES

1. Chatellier G, Zapletal E, Lemaitre D, Menard J, Degoulet P. The number needed to treat: a clinically useful nomogram in its proper context. *BMJ* 1996;321:426–429.
2. Cook RJ, Sackett DL. The number needed to treat: a clinically useful measure of treatment effect. *BMJ* 1995;310:452–454.

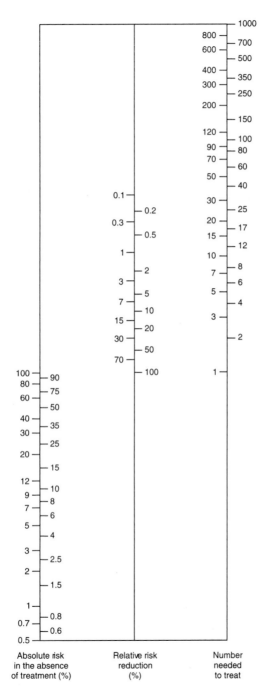

| Absolute risk in the absence of treatment (%) | Relative risk reduction (%) | Number needed to treat |

Abbreviations

AR	Absolute risk	**NS**	Not significant
ARR	Absolute risk reduction	**OR**	Odds ratio
ARI	Absolute risk increase	**P**	P value
CI	Confidence interval	**RCT**	Randomised controlled trial
CCT	Controlled clinical trial	**RR**	Relative risk
HR	Hazard ratio	**RRI**	Relative risk increase
NNH	Number needed to harm	**RRR**	Relative risk reduction
NNT	Number needed to treat	**WMD**	Weighted mean difference

How to calculate risk

AR = # events (good or bad) in treated or control groups/ # people in that group

ARC = AR of events in the control group

ART = AR of events in the treatment group

ARR = ARC − ART

RR = ART/ARC = 1 − RRR

RRR = (ARC − ART)/ARC = 1 − RR

NNT = 1/ARR

To express decimals as percentages, multiply by 100.

If:

the RR (or OR) = 1, or the CI includes 1, there is no significant difference between treatment and control groups

the RR > 1 and the CI does not include 1, events are significantly more likely in the treatment than the control group

the RR < 1 and the CI does not include 1, events are significantly less likely in the treatment than the control group

RR of 0.8 means a RRR of 20% (meaning a 20% reduction in the relative risk of the specified outcome in the treatment group compared with the control group).

RRR is usually constant across a range of absolute risks. But the ARR is higher and the NNT lower in people with higher absolute risks.

Example: If a person's AR of stroke, estimated from his age and other risk factors (see appendix 1), is 0.25 without treatment but falls to 0.20 with treatment, the ARR is 25% −20% = 5%; the RRR is (25% −20%)/25% = 20%; and the NNT is 1/0.05 = 20. In a person with an AR of stroke of only 0.025 without treatment, the same treatment will still produce a 20% RRR, but treatment will reduce her AR of stroke to 0.020, giving a much smaller ARR of 2.5% −2% = 0.5%, and a NNT of 200.